American Victorian Costume in Early Photographs

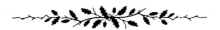

by

Priscilla Harris Dalrymple

DOVER PUBLICATIONS, INC.
New York

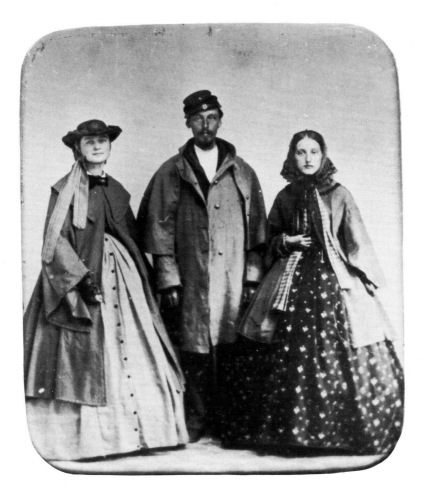

Civil War soldier, flanked by two women in hoopskirts. Their wide-sleeved cloaks are very similar to ones shown in *Peterson's Magazine* in January 1862 (pp. 10, 11, 16), as is the scarflike headdress. (Tintype.)

Copyright © 1991 by Priscilla Harris Dalrymple.
All rights reserved under Pan American and International Copyright Conventions.

Published in Canada by General Publishing Company, Ltd.,
30 Lesmill Road, Don Mills, Toronto, Ontario.
Published in the United Kingdom by Constable and Company, Ltd.,
3 The Lanchesters, 162–164 Fulham Palace Road, London W6 9ER.

American Victorian Costume in Early Photographs is a new work,
first published by Dover Publications, Inc., in 1991.

Manufactured in the United States of America
Dover Publications, Inc.
31 East 2nd Street
Mineola, N.Y. 11501

Library of Congress Cataloging-in-Publication Data

Dalrymple, Priscilla Harris.
American Victorian costumes in early photographs /
by Priscilla Harris Dalrymple.
p.   cm.
ISBN 0-486-26533-1
1. Costume—United States—History—19th century.
2. Costume—United States—History—19th century—Pictorial
works. I. Title.
GT610.D35   1991
391′.00973′09034—dc20   90-22012
CIP

Introduction

Clothing of the Victorian era, especially women's fashion, in turn delights and horrifies us. Billowing hoop skirts, modest poke bonnets, absurd and cumbersome bustles, dirt-collecting trains, painfully corseted wasp waists, leg-o'-mutton sleeves, outrageous hats—one sartorial excess succeeded another. It was the last period in the history of costume to display such incredible extravagance and impracticality in dress. Fortunately for future generations, it was also the first period that could be recorded photographically. Americans rushed to face the camera, initially being captured in daguerreotypes, then in the ambrotypes, tintypes, cartes de visite and cabinet cards that followed. From this rich legacy many images survive today, providing us with a varied and wonderful panorama of fashions and faces from the 1840s on.

From the moment the French daguerreotype process was made public in 1839, enthusiasm for photography was unquenchable. It seemed almost miraculous that an exact likeness could be obtained without paint, pencil or artist. By the middle of the year 1840 there were thriving daguerreotype galleries in Boston, New York and Philadelphia. Within a few years every city had at least one gallery, and operators penetrated many of the more rural areas in horse-drawn wagons and river barges.

Until this time, having a stylish portrait painted had generally been an indulgence only the wealthy could afford. As more daguerreotypists (often former artists who saw in photography a more lucrative field) set up shop and competition drove prices down, these new portraits became affordable to the middle class. Soon finely detailed daguerreotypes in their beautiful cases were being displayed in parlors all over the country. The idea of owning a permanent image of a friend or relative, or of achieving a semblance of immortality for oneself, was irresistible.

For the past ten years I have been collecting nineteenth-century American photographic images. Although I did not start out with any particular emphasis on costume in mind when I first began combing antique shops and flea markets, it was impossible not to become intrigued by the marvelous clothing pictured and to want to learn more about it. I found many books on the general subject, very few on the Victorian period exclusively and, to my frustration, none that was illustrated solely by American photographs.

This lacuna gradually got me thinking, as my interest and collection grew, of doing a book myself. I bought a camera for copying and made glossy black-and-white photos of over 250 images. It was surprising how contemporary and alive these men, women and children looked, once released from dark and murky tintypes, fading cartes de visite or elusive daguerreotypes. Gone was the feeling of musty age that the physical appearance of the originals sometimes evoked. The subject, not the medium, became the message. (Images 63, 88, 99, 136, 159, 188, 207 and 241 are, in fact, Canadian, but the costumes shown in them are typical of North America in general.)

The only commercial fashion illustration during this period was the engraved plate. But a type of fashion photography certainly did exist, as most of the images I have chosen indicate a very serious concern by the photographer with clothing—sometimes even to the detriment of the portrayal of the face. One has to believe that the subject was eager to have it this way, as a record of his or her fashionableness. (Why else would a lady strike a full-length profile pose in a dress with a bustle, or a man wear his top hat and overcoat for his portrait?) Such images undeniably give us a more accurate idea of how people really looked and dressed in that colorful era than fashion plates ever could.

The purpose of this book is threefold:

For the student of costume, it provides a wealth of images of ordinary Americans, as opposed to the fashion plates and photographs of royalty, statesmen and theatrical stars that generally illustrate books on this subject. (Even those priceless and delightful costumes on museum mannequins cannot fully depict the actual stance of the wearer, nor the details of expression, hairdo and accessories that are so significant.)

For the layman, it is an aid to placing family portraits in their historical context.

For the photographic historian and collector, it provides an additional tool in dating and identifying images.

Beyond this, I also hope to communicate something of the delights of collecting these special glimpses of the past. The daguerreotype and its successors have a unique power to bring the past tangibly closer to us. Going through my collection never fails to give me a deep sense of the love and hope and determination to survive that are passed on from generation to generation. Despite the fact that most of the photographers are as anonymous as their subjects, there are a number of very individualistic and appealing portrayals in the pages that follow. Suddenly these people seem real and accessible, and the nineteenth century comes alive.

Contents

The 1840s

Women's fashions have, perhaps, never been as prim and demure as they were at this time, although at evening parties the shoulders were bared expansively and the hair was often worn in bouncy corkscrew curls and adorned with flowers and other embellishments. But the typical daytime gown had a long, pointed bodice and a full, dome-shaped, floor-length skirt supported by as many as five or six petticoats. (One might be of crinoline, a stiff fabric made from flax and horsehair.) Dropped shoulders sloped into long, tight sleeves, impeding movement. Center-parted hair was pulled back severely to cover the ears, and a bun was frequently worn at the back. Sometimes hair forms were used to give great width to the sides. It took an exceptional woman to cope with all this and still look attractive. There were a few ameliorating factors, however. Bonnets, which were deep-brimmed (limiting side vision) and joined under the chin, could be very charming. Sometimes they were decorated *inside* the brim with flowers, and all sorts of other trimmings were used on the outside to good effect. Collars were of dainty lace, parasols and the fingerless black lace gloves known as "mitts" were flirtatious accessories, and capes and mantles could be worn becomingly.

Pale, muted colors were consistent with the lack of exuberance of line. *Godey's Lady's Book* describes ensembles: "pale pink and black striped gown, mantle of lace, pink roses and ribbons, pale green parasol; pink silk gown with stripes, green mantle, pale yellow bonnet; slate-blue checked silk dress, white fringed shawl, pink bonnet, green parasol"[1] and so on. The colors were more harmonious than the description would lead one to believe. Vegetable dyes were all that were available, and they produced soft, grayed tones that blended well.

In the late forties women's sleeves began to widen and skirts sometimes had flounces. The bodice was shorter and not necessarily pointed. Corsets were still an indispensable part of the wardrobe, but *Godey's* noted with satisfaction that "happily for the rising generation of young ladies, the custom of tight-lacing is comparatively little practised."[2]

Indoor caps were worn by married women and older spinsters in the house. On visits they were often carried, to be put on after the bonnet was removed, or they were simply worn under the bonnet en route. These caps, usually made by the lady herself, ranged from the simplest, plainest variety to elaborate confections of lace, ribbons and flowers that must have delighted the wearer and her admirers alike.

Little girls followed their mothers' fashions, with V-shaped vertical tucks in the bodice, dropped shoulders and tight sleeves, but their skirts were much shorter. Older girls had progressively longer skirts. White ankle-length pantalets (often lace-trimmed), white stockings and low black shoes usually completed the outfit. A girl's hair was always parted in the middle, and generally worn either in corkscrew curls or short, straight and combed behind the ears.

Small boys also wore dresses in much the same style as their sisters', or skirtlike tunics and pantalets, until they were "breeched" when the child was age four or five. Often the only clue to the sex of a child in a daguerreotype is how the hair is parted. If it is on the side, it is male. (A possible variation, for both boys and men, was to part it on both sides, and brush the center hair up, or back, into waves or curls.) Once out of skirts, boys wore pants, usually of ankle length, that buttoned to the shirt—a practical arrangement in which the buttons were simply moved down as the boy grew—and sometimes a short, simple jacket.

An undeniably charming style for little girls and boys, shown time and again in both paintings and images of the era, were wide-necked dresses that bared the neck and shoulders. At a time when houses had no central heating, and infant and child mortality was so high, one would like to think that this reckless apparel was saved for special occasions. To the contrary, there is evidence that it was frequently worn, whatever the season. It did not lack for critics, however; *Godey's* decried it as a "pernicious fashion . . . uncomfortable as well as injurious,"[3] but to no avail. Julia Dent Grant writes, "the children's arms and legs were bare in those days . . .," and she, like countless other parents, found that her child "looked very pretty with his dimpled knees and shoulders."[4]

A gentleman of the forties would wear a dark frock coat (which resembled a short, lightweight, fitted overcoat being worn indoors), trousers that had neither crease nor cuff, and a very tall top hat of silk or beaver. Practically his only chance to express some individuality lay in his choice of a waistcoat, for which figured and bright-colored fabrics were still in style. Collars were either the very high, stiff "parricide" type, with points that projected over the cheeks, or the later, turned-down style that was popular with younger men. Cravats and neckcloths were wrapped and tied in a variety of ways. Hair was parted on the side, often curled forward over the ears and worn fairly short. Sideburns were popular. Sometimes a beard was worn below the chin, but the face itself was usually clean-shaven. The aim of most men was to appear dignified and sober, and in this they certainly succeeded.

[1] *Fashions and Costumes from Godey's Lady's Book*, ed. Stella Blum (New York: Dover Publications, Inc., 1985), pp. 12–14.
[2] *Godey's Lady's Book*, vol. 35 (1848), p. 67.
[3] *Ibid.*
[4] *The Personal Memoirs of Julia Dent Grant*, (New York: G. P. Putnam's Sons, 1975), p. 74.

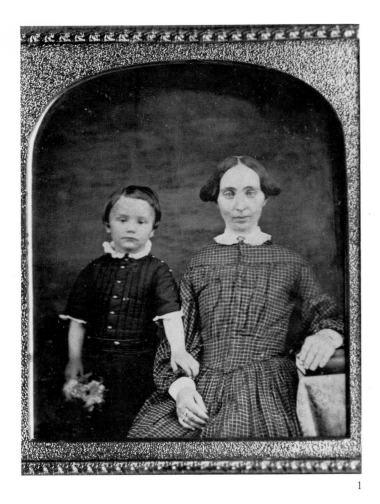

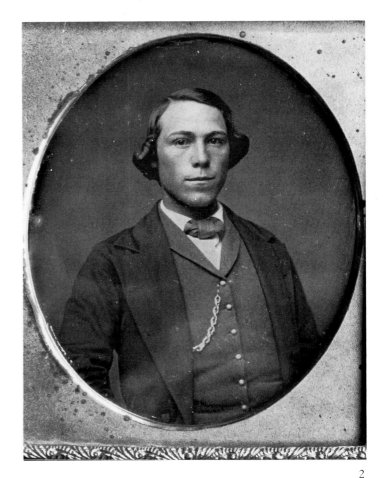

1.
A vestige of the 1830s remains in this woman's sleeve fullness; the long-waisted, vertically tucked bodice is typical of the forties, as is the hairstyle. The boy's bodice and collar echo his mother's.

2.
Gentleman with hair fashionably curled over the ears, frock coat, shawl-collared waistcoat with massive watch chain, cravat tucked under turned-down collar.

3.
Woman in silk taffeta dress with embroidered "mancherons" (short oversleeves), tight under-sleeves, boned bodice with vertical pleats. Bearded man with figured satin waistcoat.

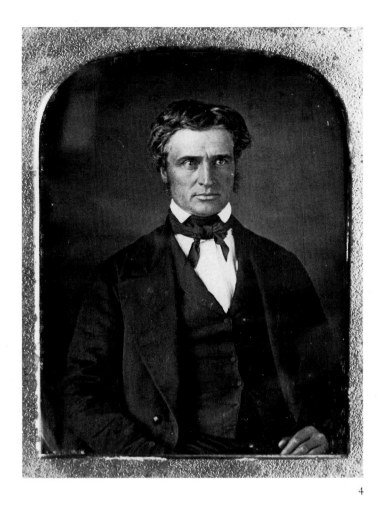

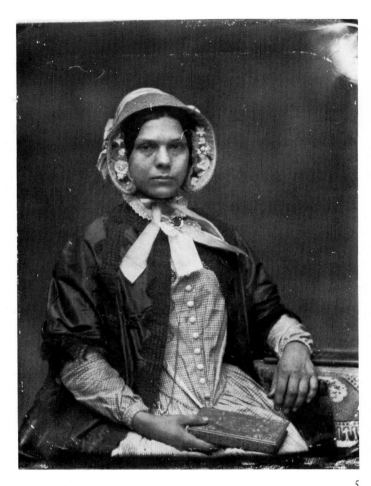

4

5

4.
Gentleman in frock coat with M-notch lapels, matching waistcoat, cravat tied in simple knot.

5.
Woman in forties straw bonnet with flowers and lace inside the brim, checked dress with pointed boned bodice and a cape-sleeved, lace-trimmed mantelet.

6.
Two girls. Corkscrew curls on the little one; the hair combed sleekly behind the ears on the older. Both have center parts—both styles that would last for decades. Dresses with vertically pleated bodices, full skirts.

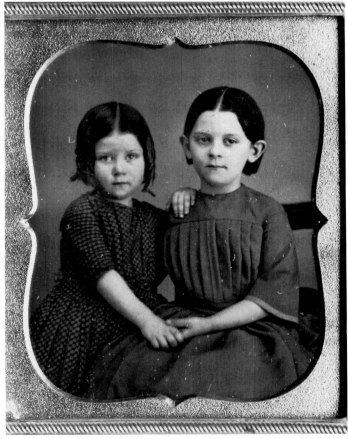

6

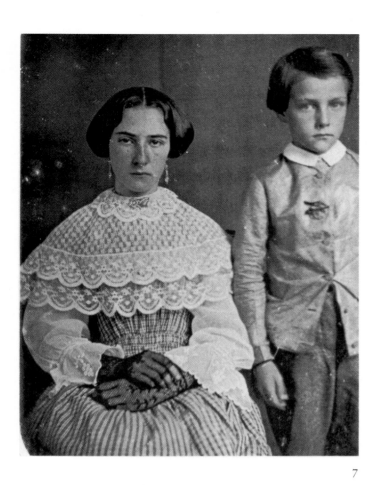

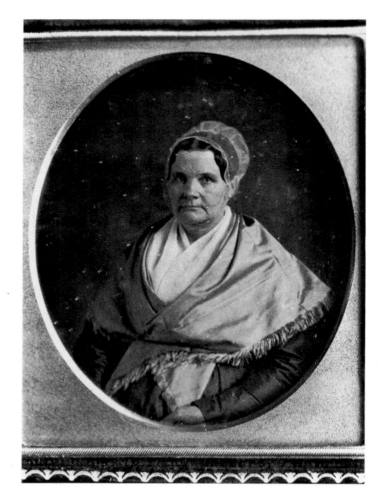

7

8

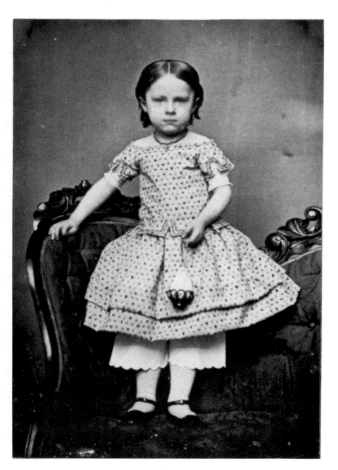

9

7.
Woman in plaid taffeta dress with filmy white work-embroidered cotton sleeves, white-net two-tiered pelerine, lace collar, brooch, earrings, mitts. The boy wears a simple, straight collarless jacket with a white shirt.

8.
This lady brings to mind Julia Grant's description of Ulysses' grandmother in 1848, "dressed in rich, dark brown . . . a snowy muslin kerchief about her shoulders, and a soft white muslin cap . . . ."[5]

9.
Little girl, standing on a Belter-style sofa, wears a patterned, short-sleeved, off-shoulder dress with a tuck in the full skirt (to allow for growth), ribbon-and-lace-trimmed undersleeves (part of her chemise), scalloped pantalets, white stockings and black slippers. She holds a reticule. Coral necklaces were worn, following the ancient tradition that held that they warded off danger.

[5]*Ibid.*, p. 57.

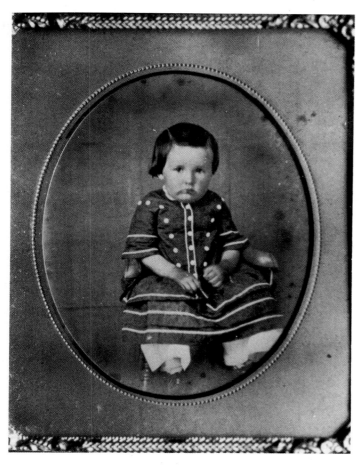

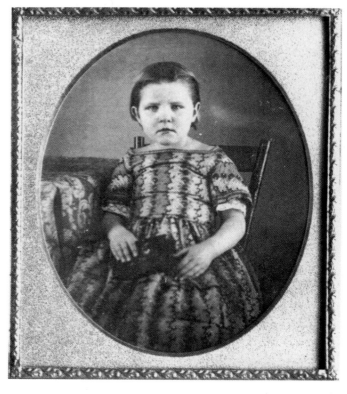

10

11

10.
Buttons and bands of piping trim this little boy's dress.

11.
Little girl in boat-necked, short-sleeved dress of floral striped material.

12.
Little boy on Gothic-Revival chair. Off-shoulder dress, vertically tucked bodice, flounces on skirt, embroidered soutache trim on sleeves and hem, pantalets with broderie anglaise scallops.

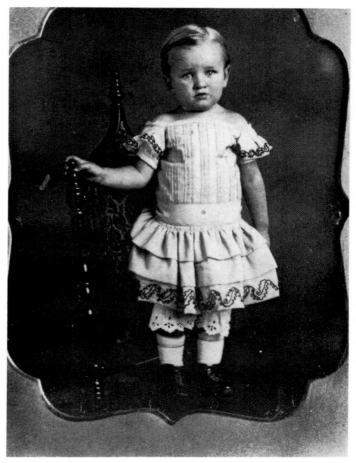

12

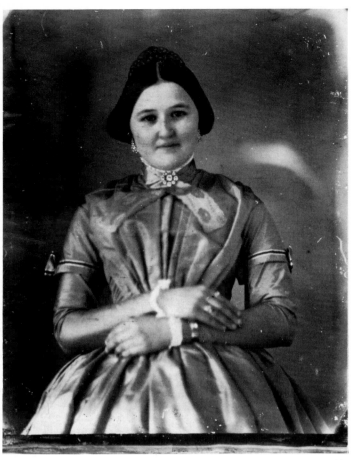

13

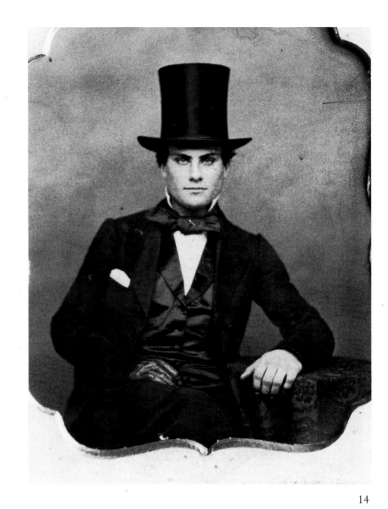

14

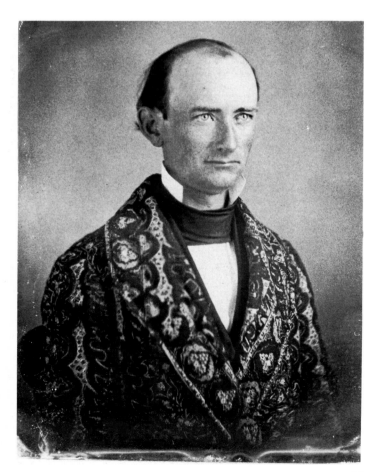

13.
Lady in silk dress with ribbon-and-bow trim, long tight sleeves, V-shaped pleated bodice, dome-shaped skirt, brooch and earrings.

14.
Man in the very tall top hat of the forties, standing collar and cravat with stickpin.

15.
Man in smoking jacket of figured velvet, standing collar, black neckcloth.

15

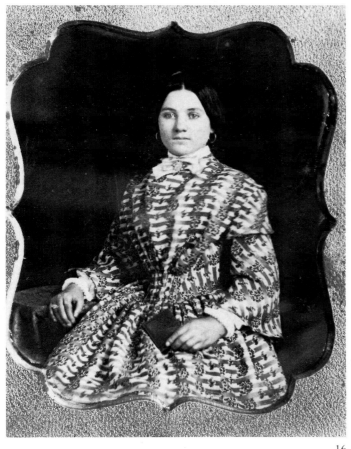

16

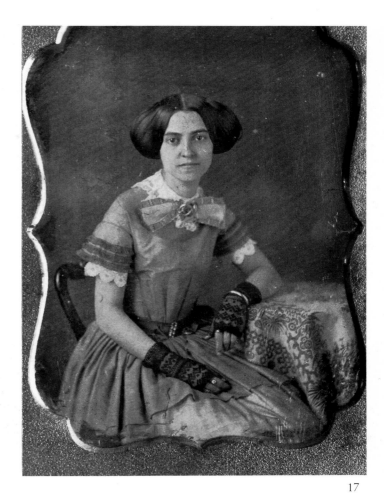

17

16.
Young woman in gown of striped and sprigged material, with the new flared sleeves of the late forties that stopped just short of the wrist to reveal a pretty white undersleeve.

17.
Fashionable woman with very full hairstyle. Gown in sheer summer fabric with dainty lace undersleeves, lace collar and ribbon with brooch; lace mitts. The ribbon belt was a fashionable option at the close of the decade.

18.
Woman with large, striped neck bow; house cap.

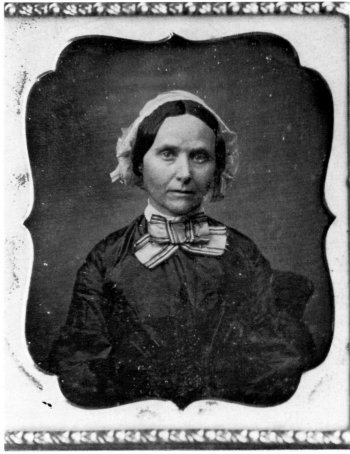

18

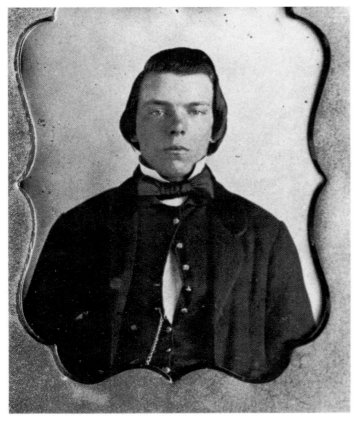

19

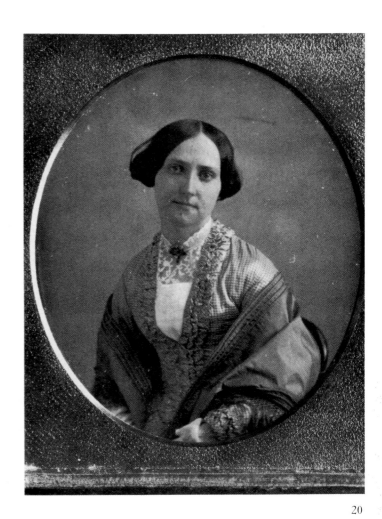

20

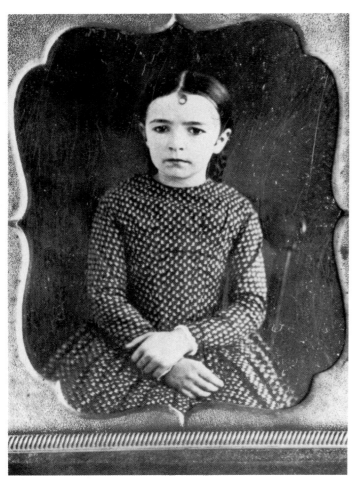

21

19.
Young man in high-cut waistcoat (the middle buttons undone), watch chain, standing collar, cravat.

20.
Lady in checked dress. The deep, ruffled V of the bodice opens over a white chemisette; silk shawl.

21.
Girl in figured dress. Tight, boned bodice, long tight sleeves, full skirt; curl in middle of forehead.

22.
Four men in frock coats, turned-down collars with wide opening filled by cravats; hair brushed forward (the man farthest left sporting two curls on top of his head).

23.
Young woman in bonnet with ruched facing, plumes and very wide "strings" (ribbons), which, said *Godey's* in 1848 (vol. 37, p. 253), were "broader than they have been for some years."

24.
Young woman in off-shoulder gown with simulated laced bodice under embroidered net overdress. The young man wears a lively-patterned waistcoat, standing collar and embroidered cravat.

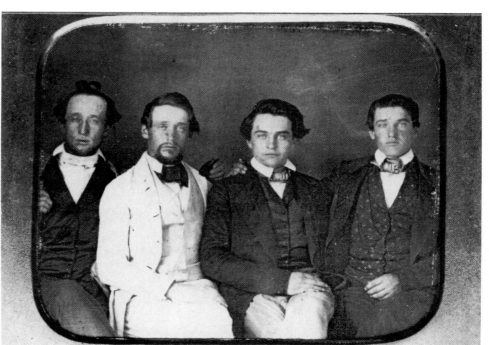

22

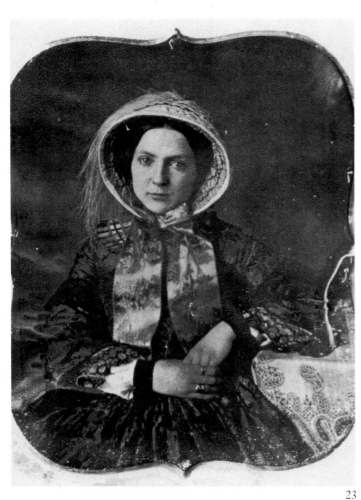

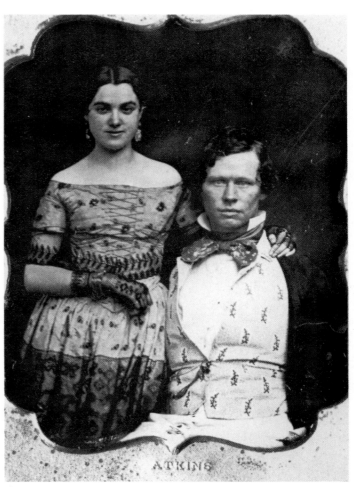

23   24

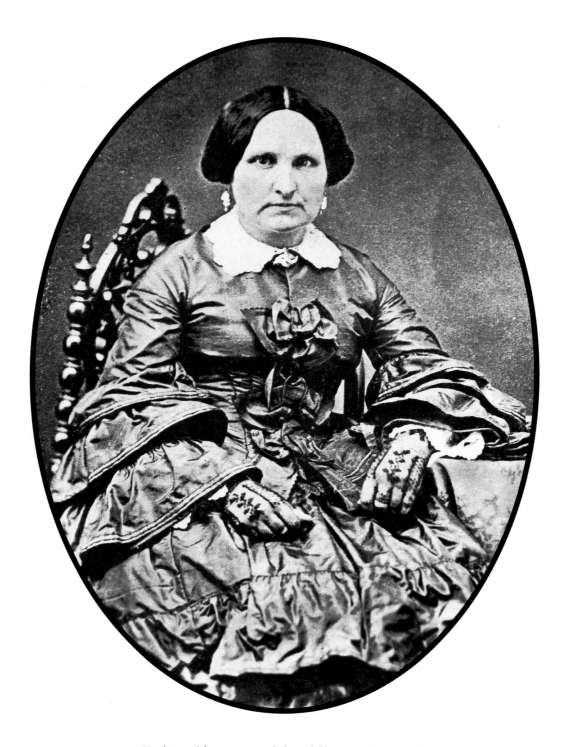

Fashionable woman of the 1850s. See Figure 37.

The 1850s

Women welcomed a marvelous innovation in the mid-fifties. Hoops of fine steel—lightweight, flexible and strong—allowed them to dispense with the heavy and cumbersome layers of petticoats previously required to maintain the shape of the skirt. Now only one petticoat was needed, the skirt over the hoops tilted and swayed provocatively with every movement and the wearer felt light and free. Admittedly, the hoops presented a few inconveniences—small pieces of furniture, for example, were often unwittingly overturned as the voluminous, ruffled, dome-shaped skirt swept by, and there was definitely a space problem on settees, carriages and pubic conveyances—but nothing stemmed the hoopskirt tide. All classes of women, except the very poorest, wore them whenever possible—and at times when it seemed quite impossible. Of a newlywed couple in a wagon train setting out on the perilous journey west, Helen Carpenter comments in her 1857 diary, "The bride wears hoops . . . we have read of hoops being worn, but they had not reached Kansas before we left. . . . Would not recommend them for this mode of traveling . . ."[1]

Fashion was important. Although under severe conditions, such as on the frontier, life was so harsh that "to get clothing sufficient to protect the body from the cold of winter and the heat of summer was the only thing thought of,"[2] in less trying circumstances most women made a valiant effort to keep up, as best they could, with the current styles, which often meant ripping apart and remaking an old dress when they could not afford a new one. In fact, in 1855, *Godey's* cautioned young women against too great a preoccupation with clothes, and chided them for frittering away their time "on flounces and opera music."[3]

Flounces were the latest trend. Some skirts had as many as 24, although three or four were more common, and the plain skirt was still amply in evidence. An already very wide skirt, if flounced, seemed even wider, making almost any waist seem small in comparison, so corsets did not have to be quite so constricting. The bodice was less elongated than in the forties. Sleeves gradually became shorter and much wider, sometimes falling in tiers and flaring out to reveal dainty white undersleeves, or "engageantes." These were often lace-and-ribbon trimmed, and were considered an article of lingerie. Lace collars were worn with a brooch, and sometimes the bodice was open to the waist to reveal a pretty chemisette.

Dresses were frequently made with two interchangeable bodices—one for day wear and the other, with a low neckline and usually a wide bertha, for dressy evening events. The revival of the French court, and the influence of the beautiful and fashionable Empress Eugénie, sparked a new emphasis on rich fabrics and lavish trim, which American fashion plates (predominantly of French origin) were quick to illustrate. However, *Godey's* took care to reassure those of its readers who considered anything French slightly immoral that the magazine had engaged an artist "to reform the foreign fashions, as far as health and delicacy require."[4] Nevertheless, the whole look was one of greater luxury and extravagance.

Bonnets were smaller and moved toward the back of the head as the decade progressed. Wide-brimmed straw hats were also worn in summer for informal occasions. Shawls, cloaks, capes and even the hooded burnoose were worn as outer garments, plus various fitted and semifitted coats—all of which had to be constructed with the tremendous spread of the hoopskirt in mind.

A few brave women, led by Amelia Bloomer, tried unsuccessfully to popularize a more practical garment—a calf-length, hoopless dress worn with long Turkish trousers. The name "bloomer" found a niche not in trousers, but in gymnastic outfits that had a full, pleated leg, tight at the bottom or at or above the knee. Mrs. Bloomer's concept failed completely to be accepted as everyday wear. A contemporary writer refers in horror to women who sink "down to the lowest depth of bloomerism, smoking, and talking slang."[5] A lady simply would have no part of it.

For men, frock coats and top hats continued to be worn much of the time. Coat, waistcoat and trousers began to match and a variety of coats became available—short, double-breasted or loose. Straw hats became acceptable in town, and a low-crowned, wide-brimmed hat called a "wide-awake" was introduced. There was considerable variety and exuberance in neckwear—cravats might be modest or flamboyant, and bow ties were popular. Fancy vests—figured or dotted satin among the most popular—also added verve to the scene. High collars were very much in evidence despite the fact that turned-down collars were more up-to-date. Full beards began to be seen now and then. Coat collars and lapels decreased in size, and braid trim was sometimes used on coat and trousers. It was becoming fashionable to button only the top button of the coat. Trousers remained creaseless and cuffless.

Dresses for little girls and boys, frequently in plaids or checks, now had somewhat shorter skirts and less vertical emphasis in the bodice, and the accompanying pantalets were also more abbreviated. Some of the time, girls wore hoops under their skirts like their mothers. Once breeched, boys frequently wore Zouave or bolero jackets with shirts buttoning to contrasting fly-front trousers. Plaid stockings and low boots were a popular novelty for both sexes, as was the use of braid trim and tassels in boys' outfits. Hair styles remained the same as in the forties.

[1] *Women's Diaries of the Westward Journey*, Lillian Schlissel (New York: Schocken Books, 1982), p. 125.
[2] *Pioneer Women: Voices From the Kansas Frontier*, Joanna L. Stratton (New York: Simon & Schuster, 1981), p. 68.
[3] *Godey's Lady's Book*, vol. L, 1855, p. 172.
[4] *Godey's Lady's Book*, vol. XXVI, 1843, p. 58.
[5] *A Woman's Thoughts About Women*, anonymous (Leipzig, 1860), p. 17.

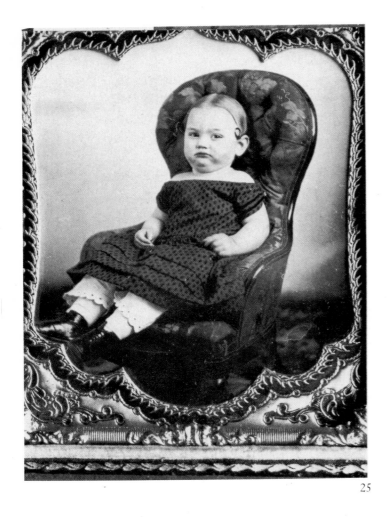

25

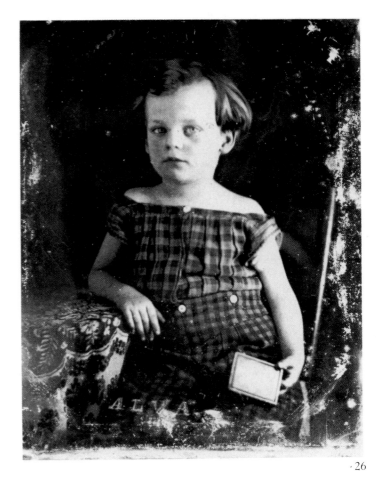

26

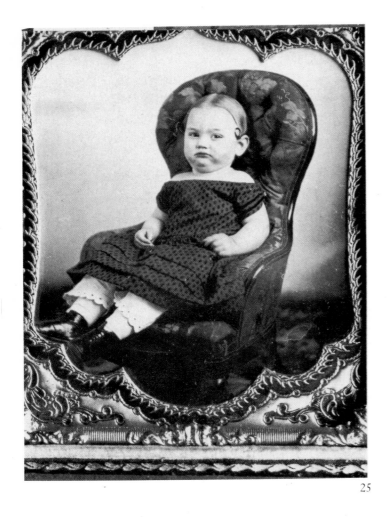

27

25.
Little girl in off-shoulder figured dress with horizontal tucks in skirt, scalloped pantalets, slicked-back hair with curl at temple.

26.
Small boy in a vertically pleated, checked, off-shoulder top that buttons to pants in a smaller check.

27.
Lady in wide-necked gown with very tight, pointed bodice; lace edging on sleeves and velvet ribbons at wrists and throat. Elaborate coiffure with V part and bare ears.

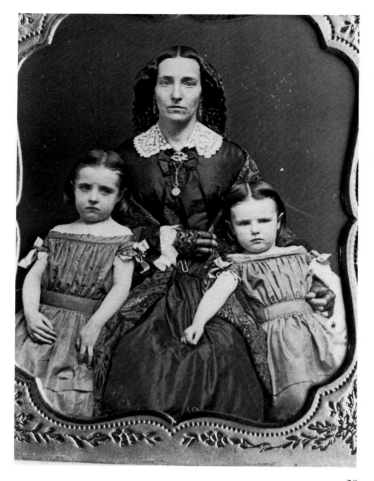

28

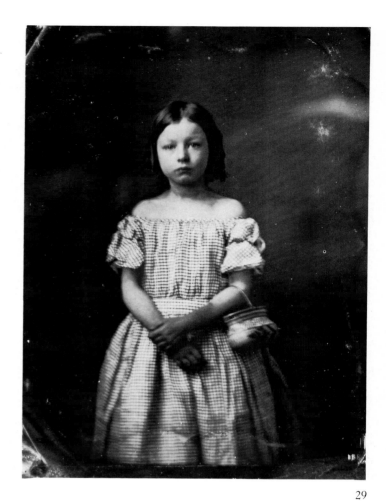

29

28.
Woman with lace collar and lace undersleeves. Little girls in matching off-shoulder dresses with vertically pleated bodices and bows on the sleeves.

29.
Girl in checked off-shoulder dress with double-puffed sleeves and basket over arm.

30.
Lady wearing bonnet with "spaniel" curls inside brim, V part, scalloped double collar, mantle and gloves.

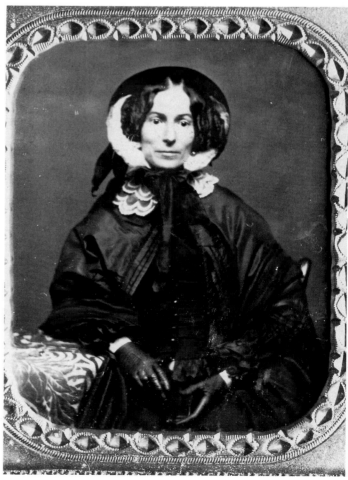

30

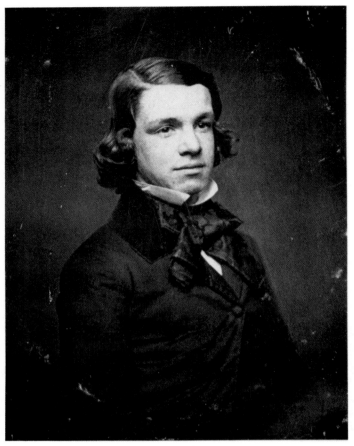

31

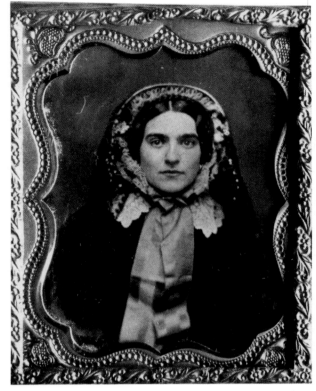

32

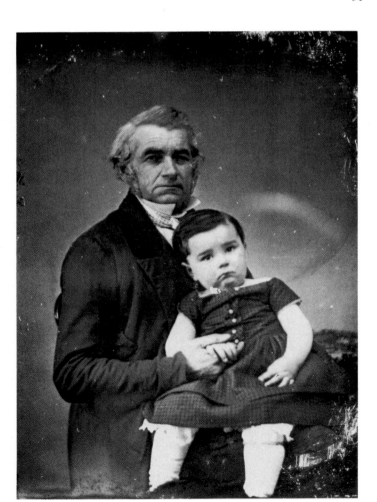

33

31.
Young man with high collar and figured satin cravat tied in a large, loose bow. In the late fifties, it began to be fashionable to fasten only the top button of the coat.

32.
Woman in bonnet with flowers and lace inside the brim, black veil and very wide ribbons.

33.
Man in frock coat, high collar and dotted cravat. Little boy in checked off-shoulder dress.

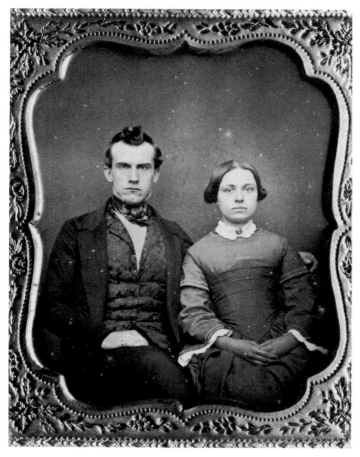

34

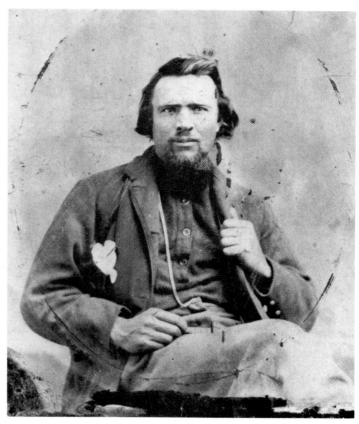

35

34.
Man in brocaded satin waistcoat, his hair in a curly mound on top of his head. The woman wears flaring, shorter sleeves, but still has pointed, rigidly boned bodice of the previous decade.

35.
Man in typical nineteenth-century wool workshirt that buttons only partway down the front.

36.
Young woman in off-shoulder print dress with flared short sleeves, loose bodice and full skirt; lace mitts.

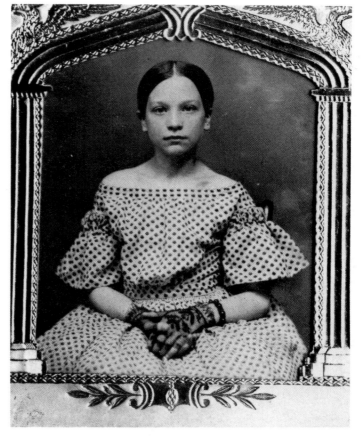

36

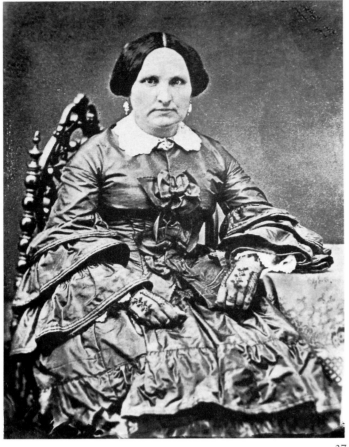

37

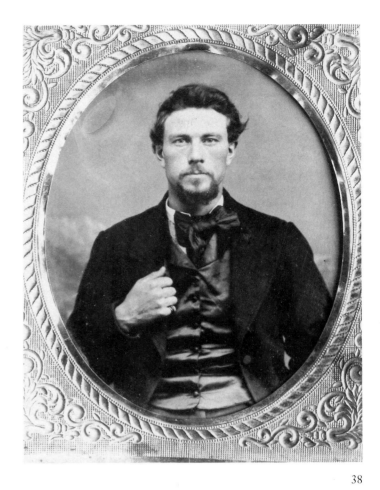

38

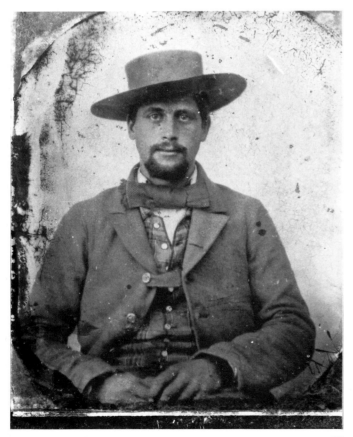

39

37.
A silk taffeta dress with pagoda sleeves with triple tiers of widely flaring flounces and a flounced skirt place this lady in the mainstream of fashion in the late fifties.

38.
Gentleman in satin waistcoat and cravat tied in a loose bow.

39.
Man in wide-brimmed, flat-crowned hat, worn tilted; partial beard and mustache; wide bow tie with fringe at one end, plaid waistcoat and coat with tab fastening.

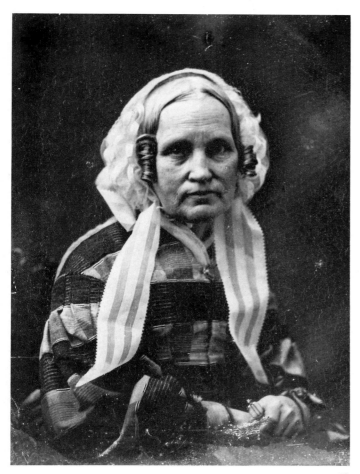

40

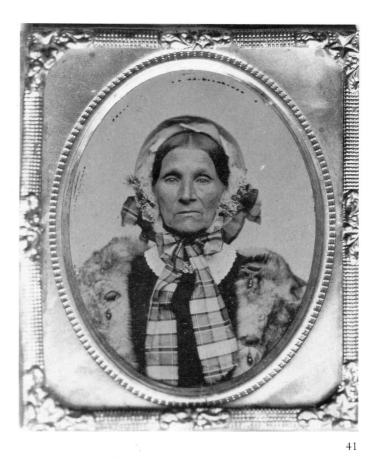

41

40.
Older woman with one large curl at either temple, wearing a net-and-ribbon house cap with long picot-edged lappets. (These hanging ribbons were purely decorative and never tied.) Full-sleeved gown of rich striped material.

41.
Woman in off-face bonnet decorated with tulle, lace, flowers and ribbon; wide plaid "strings"; fur cape.

42.
The matching cape of this striped taffeta gown gives horizontal emphasis to the bodice; wide sleeves with white undersleeves; headdress with long ribbons; hoop skirt.

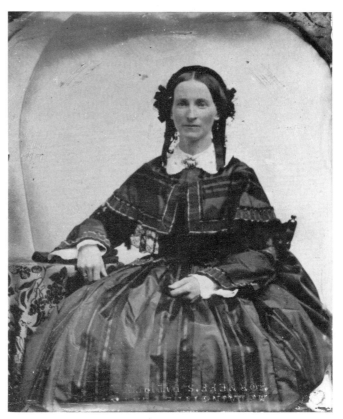

42

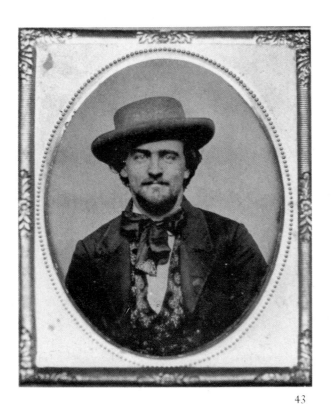

43

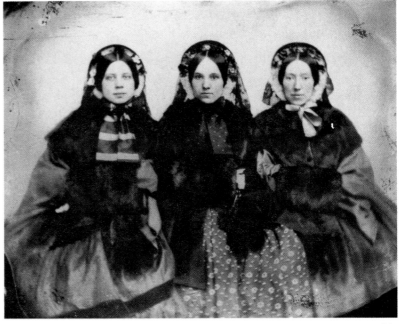

44

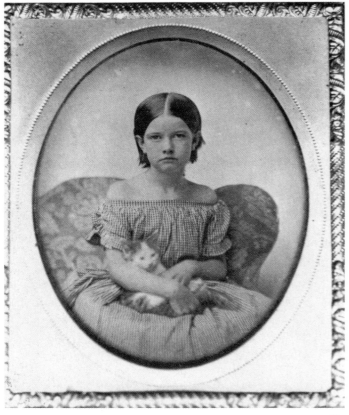

45

43.
Gentleman in low-crowned, wide-brimmed hat, figured satin waistcoat, and fancy satin tie with patterned end.

44.
Surely a mother and daughters, all dressed to the nines in the off-the-face bonnets of the fifties, with floral trim inside the brims and exceptionally wide ribbons, fur muffs, fur tippets and hoopskirts.

45.
Typical off-shoulder checked dress and hairstyle.

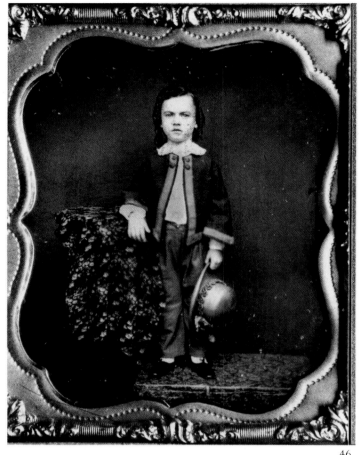

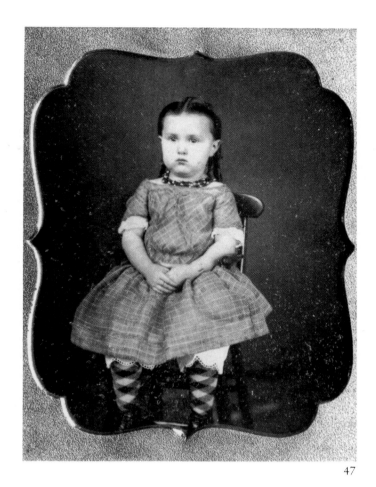

46

47

46.
A boy with long curls wears a loose jacket with wide ribbon trim, lace collar and peg-top trousers, and holds a wide-brimmed hat with decoration around base of crown.

47.
Plaid stockings were the latest fashion. This little girl wears them with a checked dress, beads and scalloped pantalets.

48.
Little boy with unruly hair in very short dress with soutache embroidery and a great expanse of rumpled pantalets below.

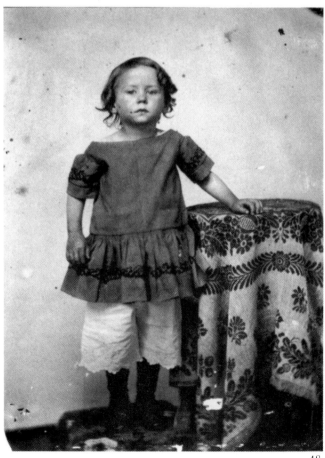

48

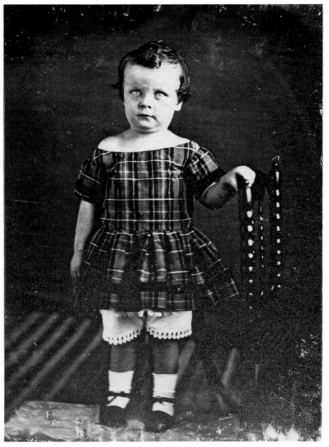

49

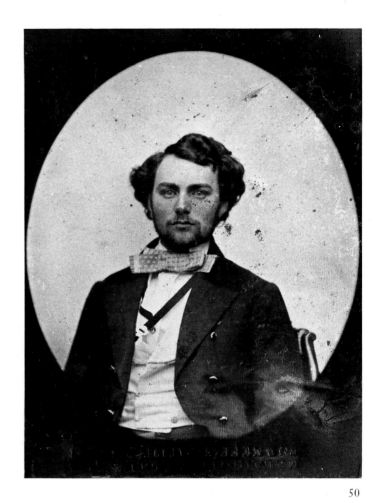

50

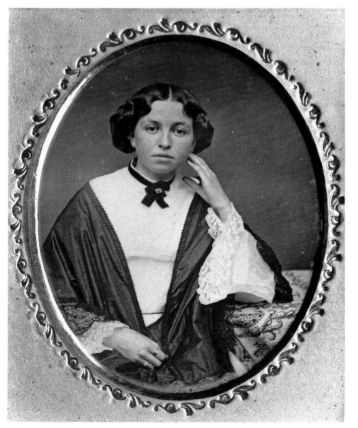

51

49.
Small boy in plaid dress with pantalets, white ankle socks and low black shoes. His hair is curled on top and brushed forward at the sides.

50.
Young man with big, checked bow tie with fringe on one end; double-breasted waistcoat; double-breasted frock coat.

51.
Woman with very wide lace-trimmed sleeves; ribbon bow at neck; lace-trimmed shawl.

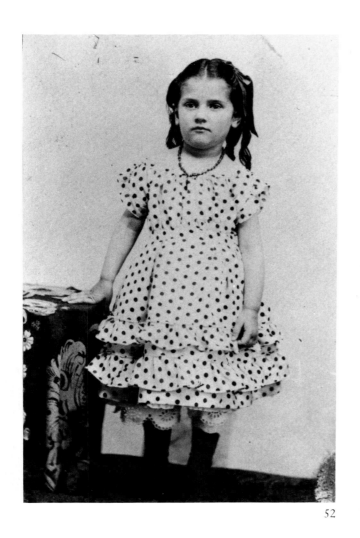

52

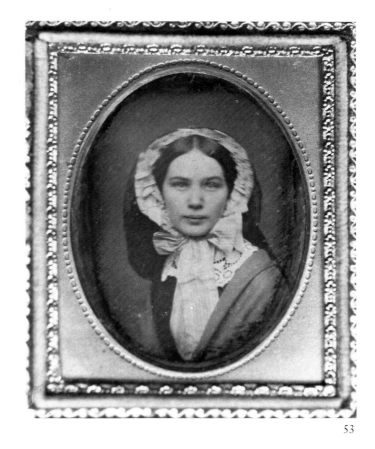

53

52.
Girl in polka-dot dress with flounces; pantalets with broderie anglaise edging; coral necklace.

53.
Young woman in hood tied with large bow; lace collar.

54.
Two men with beards and wide bow ties; one wears a figured vest.

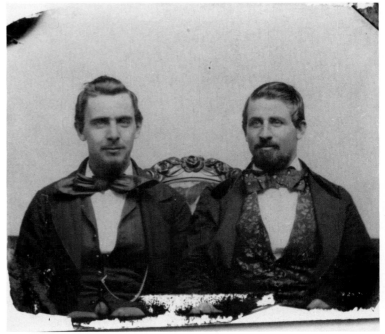

54

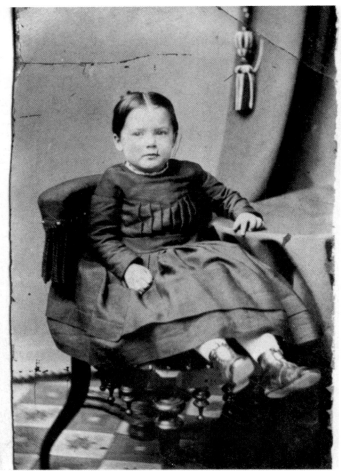

55

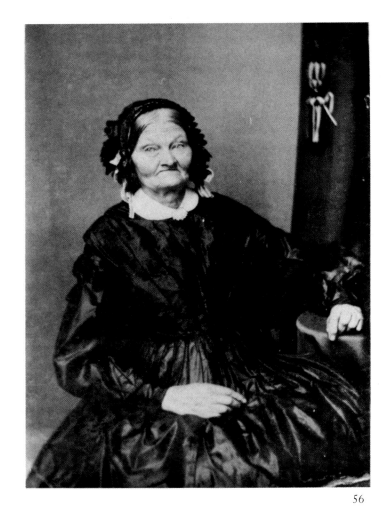

56

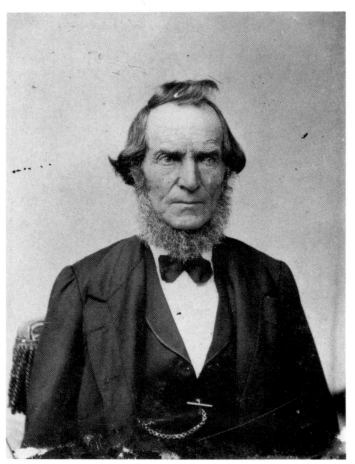

57

55.
Little girl in drop-shouldered, long-sleeved, full-skirted dress with pleated bodice; white stockings and high shoes.

56.
Older lady (perhaps grandmother of No. 55—notice same background) in dress reminiscent of the forties, with pleats fanning outward from waist to shoulder; headdress with ribbons and lace.

57.
Older gentleman in frock coat, small bow tie, saucer or trencher beard, hair brushed down on sides and swept up on top.

The 1860s

Hoopskirt mania continued unabated in the early sixties, war or no war. For evening wear skirts could measure as much as five or more yards around at the hem, but by the middle of the decade, the front of the gown was flattening out somewhat, with the greatest fullness moving toward the back. A lady wearing a cape or cloak and a little "spoon" bonnet on the back of her head, its brim pointing heavenward, presented a peculiarly triangular appearance. Flounces disappeared, leaving skirts plain or decorated with applied trim in a geometric pattern. The sewing machine, invented in the forties but just beginning to have an impact, made this kind of work much easier for those who could afford it. Wide sleeves were still worn, but began to give way to more moderate styles such as the bishop sleeve, full but tight at the cuff. Pointed bodices were being supplanted by shorter, rounder ones, worn with belts.

Separates provided a means of being resourceful as well as fashionable. A beautiful and economical style, according to *Peterson's Magazine* in 1862, was the full-sleeved Garibaldi shirt (inspired by the immense popularity of this champion of Italian freedom) which "will answer to wear with two or three old dress skirts, after the bodies are no longer fit for use."[1] The various short jackets currently in vogue, such as the Zouave, could serve the same purpose, "enabling a lady to give greater variety to her costume, without being extravagant."[2]

A refreshing addition to the scene, as the decade progressed, was the ankle-length dress—albeit still worn with hoops. This outfit was intended for such activities as walking, archery, croquet and ice-skating, the last-named so universally enjoyed that one newspaper referred to it as "our national winter exercise."[3] An 1860 Winslow Homer engraving shows ladies having to hold up their long skirts by hand while ice-skating; in a similar Homer scene, executed six years later, not only are they skating vigorously in shorter skirts that need no lifting, but in the background a game of crack-the-whip is in progress, with the lady on the end about to be spun off on a wild trip across the ice.

In the second half of the sixties dresses began to be more elaborately decorated. Ruffles, pleats, scallops, fringe and buttons were popular. Skirts, except for sport, remained floor-length and sometimes had trains. The hoopskirt grew smaller, and peplums or overskirts became an essential part of the costume, showing an increasing tendency to be pulled up and gathered toward the back, an effect that was often heightened by a sash with a large bow. By the end of the decade, this emphasis on the rear of the gown had developed into a true bustle, with its own artifical support, and the enormous hoopskirt was only a memory.

The bonnet no longer reigned supreme. Small hats were now perched on the top of the head, and little pillbox hats were worn at a rakish angle on the forehead, leaving room for an increasingly large chignon at the back, often enclosed in a decorative snood. Wide-brimmed straw hats were seen in summer. As the decade progressed, masses of false hair were added and curls might be worn on the forehead. Eventually quite elaborate hairdos, complete with two or three very long sausage curls hanging down over one shoulder, were stylish.

Now and then the bonnet still proved to be more than mere decoration. Julia Grant tells about an incident during the Civil War when she and various other members of Lincoln and Grant's entourage were on the James River in Admiral Porter's gig (an open longboat) in a supposedly safe area. Suddenly the alarming news came that Confederate sharpshooters had been spotted on the shore and had them within rifle range. The admiral immediately reassured his nervous passengers and crew that, despite this, they were in no actual danger. "These Southern fellows are all too gallant. They would not fire on a boat with women in it. These ladies' bonnets will protect us."[4]

The masculine silhouette finally showed some ripples of change, becoming less close-fitting and shapely. Two new styles introduced in the late fifties slowly began to take hold. One was the suit, with coat, trousers and waistcoat (or sometimes just two of these elements) matching. The other was the sack coat, boxy in cut, with no waist seam and a rather bulky sleeve. Both were appropriate for informal wear. Plaid and checked trousers were fashionable. Frock coats and top hats were still very much on the scene. Beards were becoming more common, as were turned-down collars and narrow bow ties, although there was no general uniformity. For example, a photograph of the class of 1860 at Union College, Schenectady, shows 11 men and 11 different styles of hair, collars and ties!

Girls' clothes continued to follow the basic trends of women's fashions. One popular outfit was the Garibaldi shirt worn with a full skirt that had a wide band of contrasting-color material near the hem. There were also "high" and "low" Garibaldi dresses (a reference to the neckline) that were cut along the same lines. Boys, too, wore the shirt with full Garibaldi pants, cut off below the knee either straight or like knickers. Military-type caps and capes were frequently seen. Horizontally striped stockings and boots were popular. Hairstyles for both sexes were similar to those of the previous decade, and little children continued to be dressed alike until the boys were breeched at around four or five years.

[1] *Peterson's Magazine*, vol. 41, Jan. 1862, p. 96.
[2] *Ibid.*, vol. 42, Dec. 1862, p. 469.
[3] *Frank Leslie's Illustrated Newspaper*, Jan. 13, 1866.
[4] Grant, *op. cit.*, p. 148.

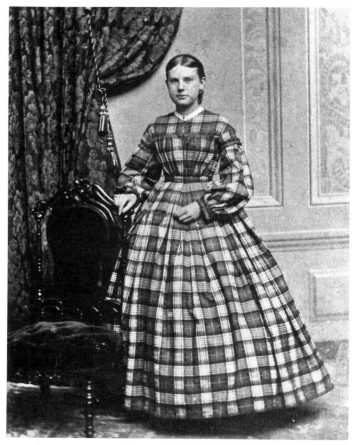

58

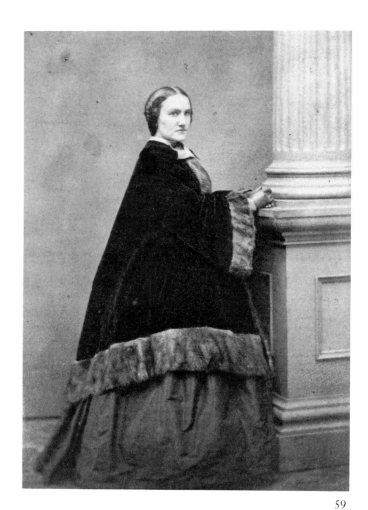

59

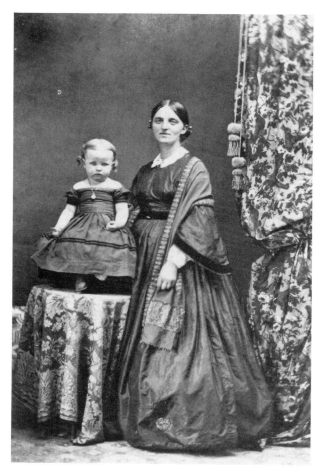

60

58.
Young woman in plaid gown with hoopskirt; full sleeves gathered at wrist; center-parted hair pulled back, with ears exposed.

59.
A fur-trimmed velvet sacque with flaring sleeves, worn over a hoopskirt.

60.
Woman in dress with belt, hoopskirt and pagoda sleeves (which soon would go out of style). Little girl bare-shouldered and also in hoopskirt.

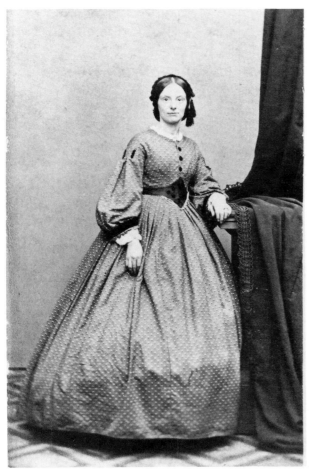

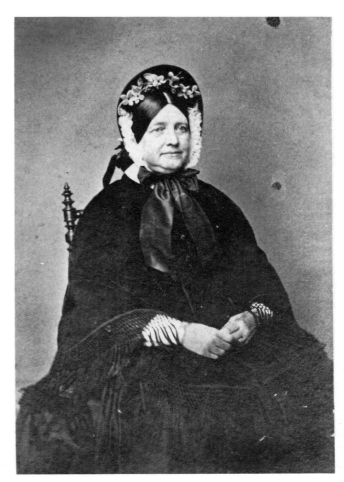

61

62

61.
A diamond-shaped "Swiss" belt is worn with a
dotted-Swiss gown with bishop sleeves; house cap
with tassels. (The hoop in the skirt is clearly
visible—a solecism.)

62.
"Mrs. Poole." An off-face bonnet with flowers
inside the brim at the crown; net trim on the sides;
fringed shawl.

63.
Epaulets and similarly trimmed triangular
applied pieces on the lower arm add sleeve interest
to this belted dress, and reflect the strong military
feeling created by the Civil War.

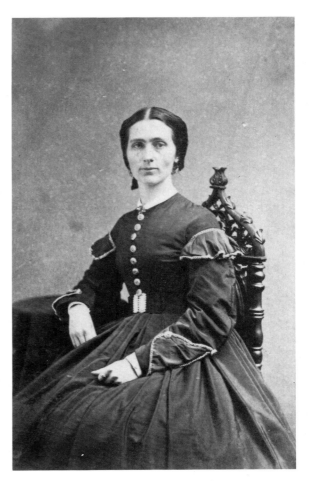

63

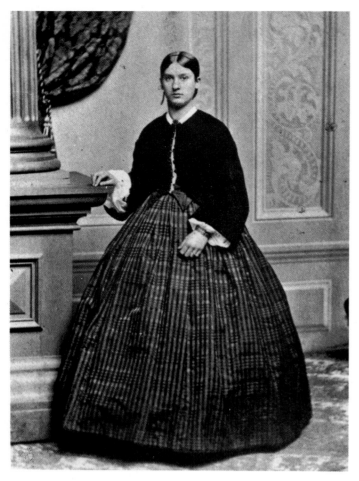

64

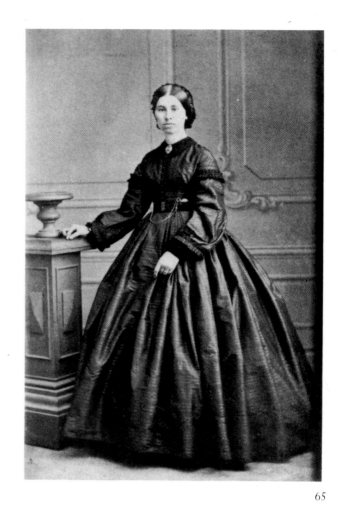

65

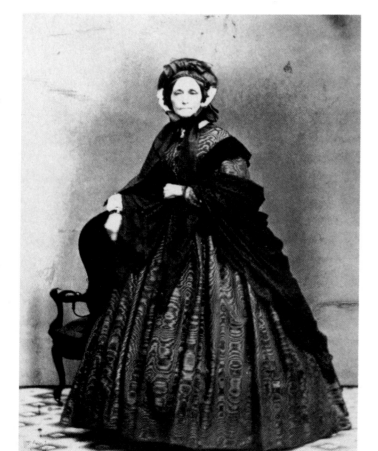

66

64.
Bolero-type jackets were now fashionable. This one is worn with a voluminous plaid hoopskirt.

65.
"For deep mourning . . . black collars and sleeves are indispensable," said *Peterson's Magazine* in May 1862, p. 426. This young woman may well be a Civil War widow. Note the watch tucked into the belt of her handsome gown.

66.
An elegant moiré gown with a sweeping hoopskirt; black lace shawl; bonnet.

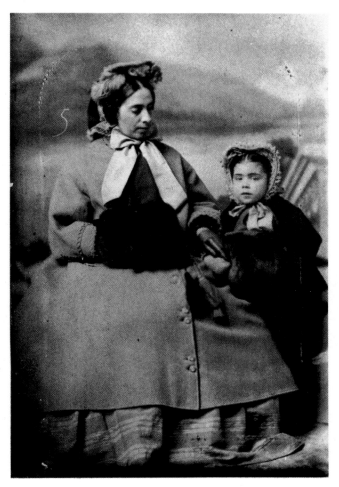

67

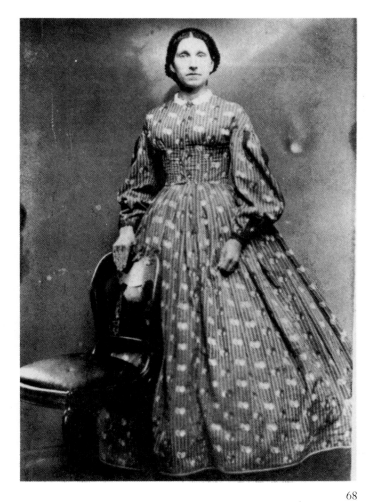

68

67.
There could be no skimping on material if a coat was to accommodate a hoopskirt. This lady wears a very small bonnet with plumes; the little girl's bonnet is heart-shaped. Both carry fur muffs.

68.
Woman in vertically striped gown with floral pattern; bishop sleeves; hoopskirt.

69.
A diamond-patterned gown with double ruffles at the shoulder and unusually tight sleeves; the hoopskirt is so wide it cannot be encompassed by the photograph.

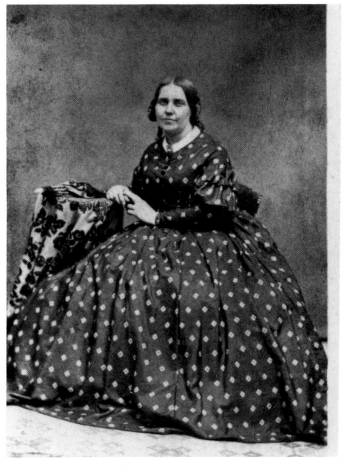

69

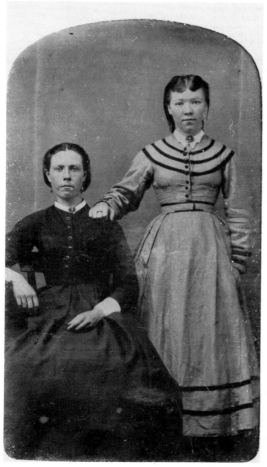

70

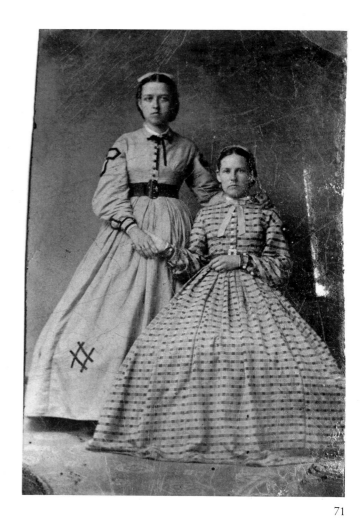

71

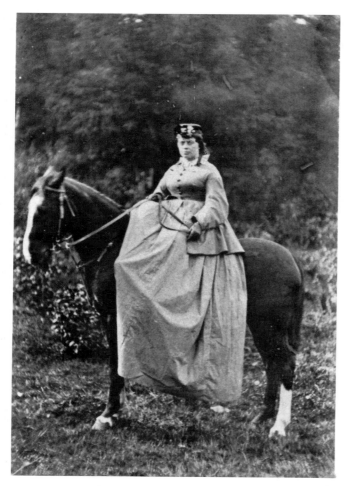

72

70.
Probably a mother and daughter, the latter, right, in ill-fitting gown with rather wavering bands of ribbon trim.

71.
Applied geometric decoration on the younger woman's dress. Both ladies in hoopskirts with wide belts; typical hairdos.

72.
Lady on horseback in a sidesaddle riding habit, 1864–66.

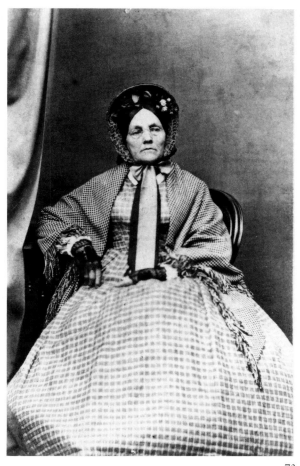

73

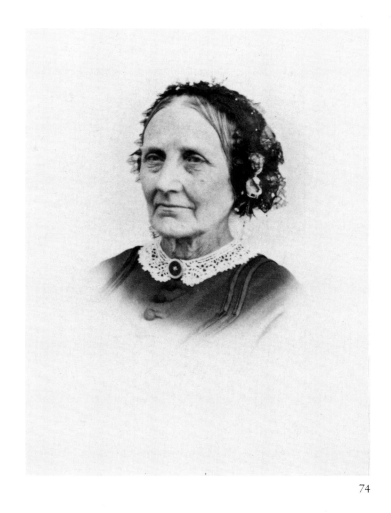

74

73.
Older lady wearing spectacles. Checked gown worn with shawl of finer checks; black lace mitts; bonnet with interior trim; hoopskirt.

74.
Older lady in dainty house cap of lace and flowers; crocheted collar; small brooch.

75.
Woman with corkscrew curls, holding two children in similar dresses having parallel bands of contrasting trim.

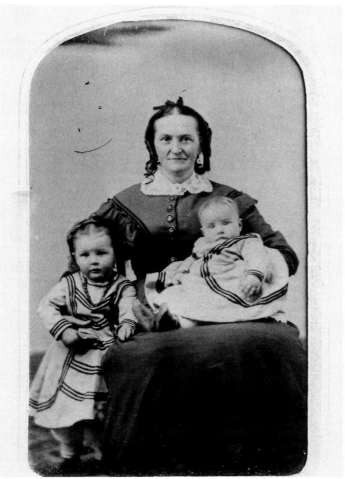

75

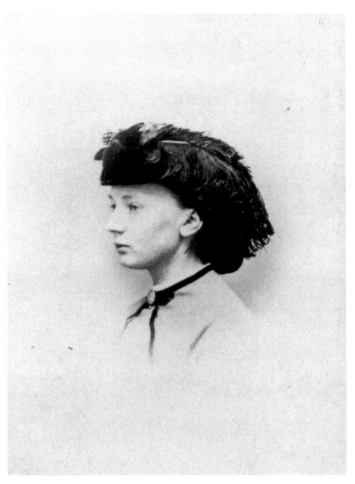

76

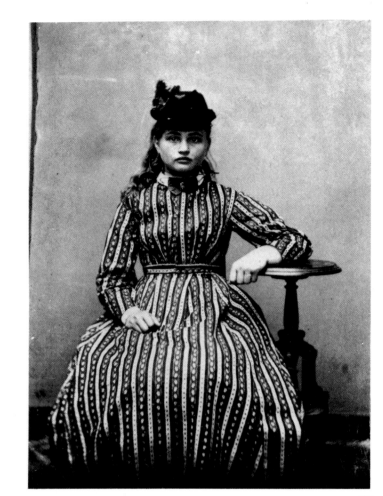

77

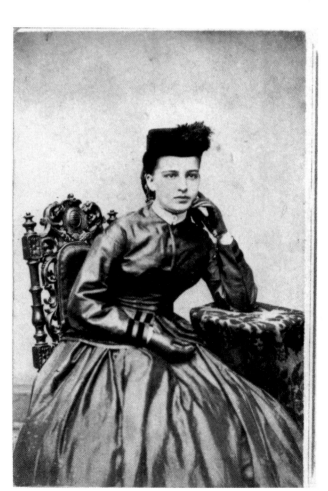

78

76.
A plumed jockey hat, worn on the forehead; hair in snood; ca. 1864–66.

77.
Young woman in striped dress; small hat worn forward; shoulder-length curly hair.

78.
Pillbox hat; lustrous silk taffeta gown; leather gloves.

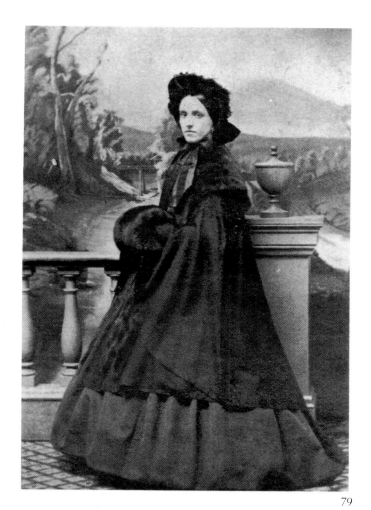

79

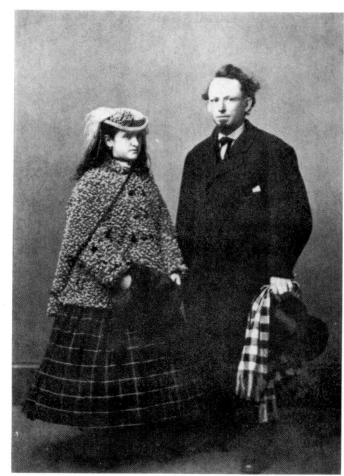

80

79.
"Dec 1862." Flattened or oval hoopskirt; cloak with fur collar and muff; spoon bonnet with bavolet concealing back hair.

80.
The woman wears a windowpane-checked, hooped walking-length short skirt, bouclé jacket and muff and a little hat with a plume that hangs down over her long hair. The man wears an overcoat and carries a boldly checked scarf and top hat.

81.
A bearded man in a low-crowned hat stands behind two ladies, both of whom wear jaunty hats tilted forward to allow for a chignon behind. The two long corkscrew curls were very fashionable in the late sixties. Paisley-type shawl and flounced plaid dress on left; fur-trimmed cloak on right.

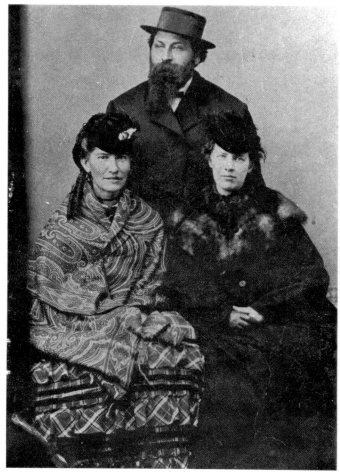

81

The 1860s ❧ 31

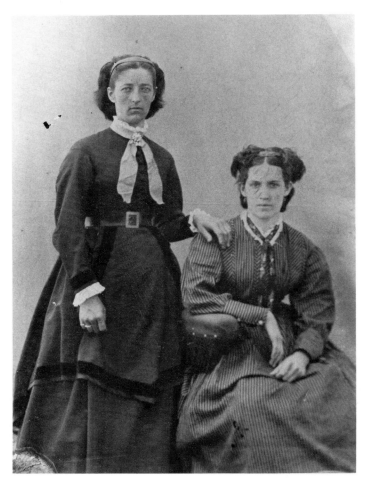

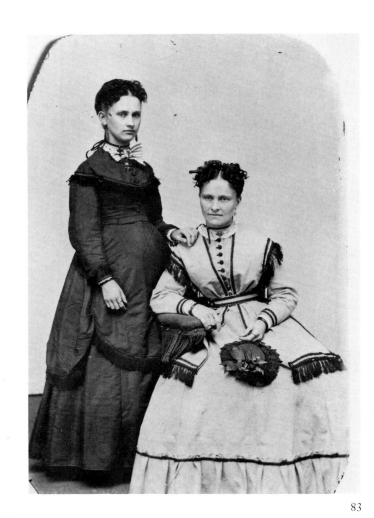

82

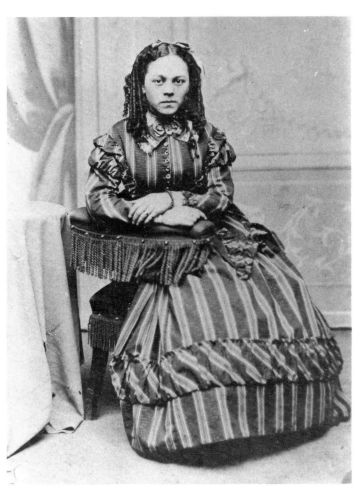

84

82.
On the left, a young woman in dress with over-skirt, her short hair pulled back with a headband. The fullness toward the temples on the young woman on the right was a short-lived trend, and the windblown look certainly accidental.

83.
The young woman on the left, who appears to be pregnant, wears a dress with the fashionable overskirt of the late sixties. Both ladies display considerable amounts of the fringe that was popular at the time.

84.
Young woman in striped dress, with the same fabric used on the bias for trim. Her corkscrew curls are a little old-fashioned.

83

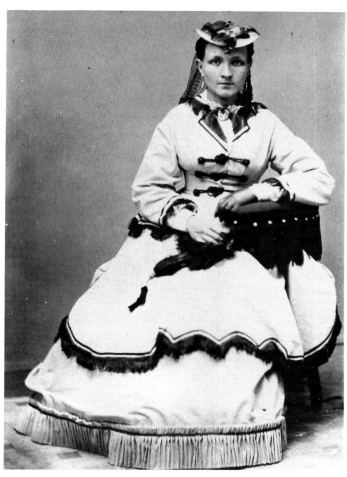

85

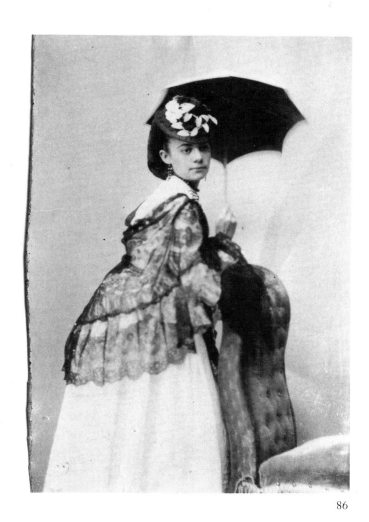

86

85.
Woman in gown with pleated hem; scalloped and fringed overskirt; frog closures on bodice; pancake hat with veil; folding parasol.

86.
The "Grecian Bend" was a stance affected by some up-to-the-minute ladies during a brief period in the late sixties. This lady wears a lace shawl, tiny hat and pendant earrings. Her hair is in a snood, and she holds an open parasol.

87.
An end-of-the-decade gown with pleats, bows and a ruffled overskirt; heavy chain necklace; bow and brooch at throat; earrings. At the end of the decade, a good deal of jewelry was worn.

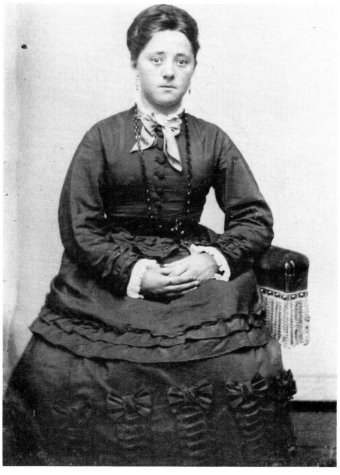

87

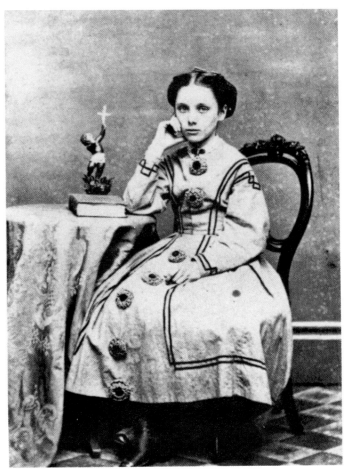

88

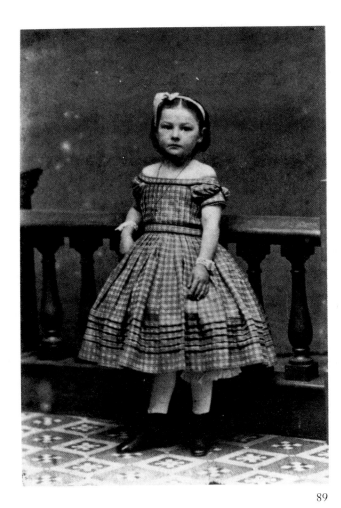

89

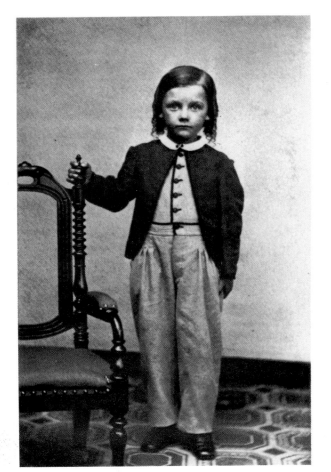

90

88.
Teenage girl in almost-grown-up-length dress with applied geometric decoration and large rosettes up the front.

89.
Little girl in short-sleeved off-shoulder dress, hoopskirt, pantalets, white stockings, black boots, hair ribbon and ribbon bracelets.

90.
Boy with curls; short jacket; braid-trimmed shirt buttoning to peg-top trousers.

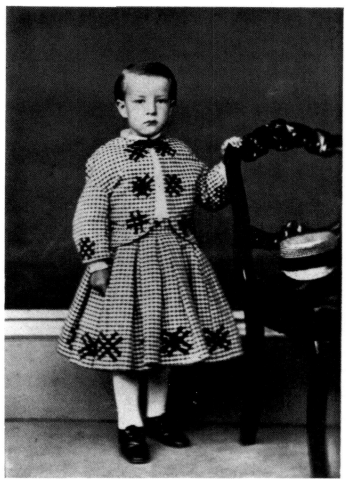

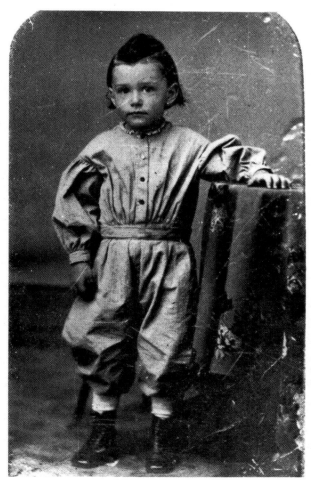

91

92

91.
Boy in checked jacket and full skirt with applied geometric trim; white stockings; low black shoes; short hair.

92.
Little boy in drop-shouldered, full-sleeved blouse of finely checked material, with matching baggy Garibaldi-type pants. Necklace is probably coral. Hair parted on both sides, and piled up in the middle.

93.
"December 12, 1861." The older boy's drop-shouldered top buttons to full-length trousers; the younger is in a dress with wide bands of dark trim; pantalets.

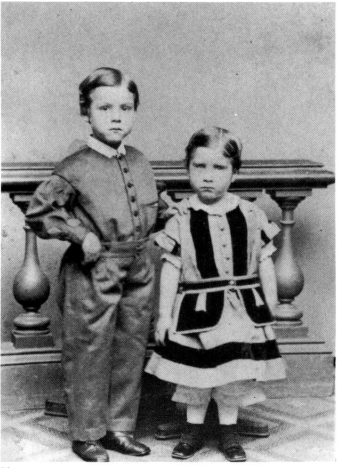

93

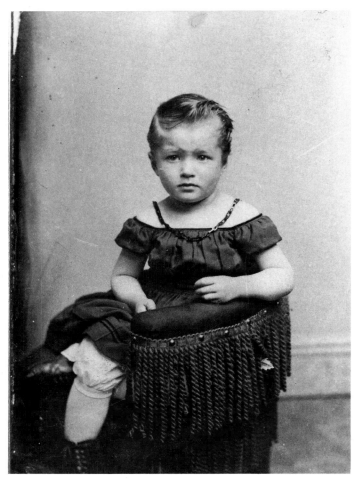

94

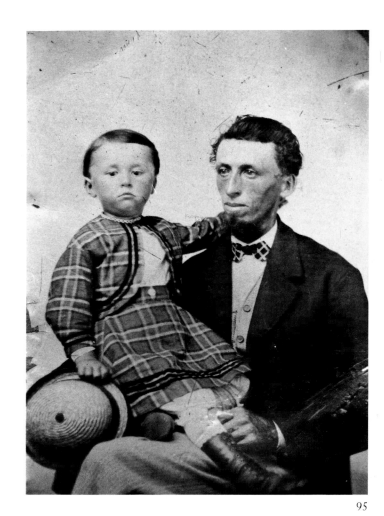

95

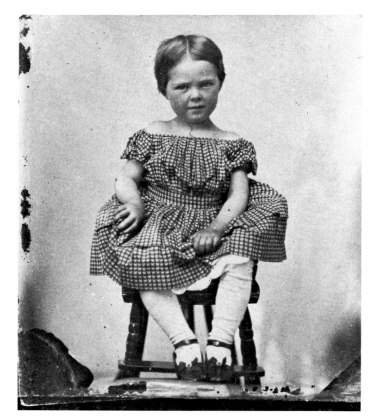

96

94.
Small boy in off-shoulder dress, tightly cuffed pantalets and a heavy chain necklace such as ladies wore.

95.
A boy in plaid bolero jacket and matching button-on skirt holds his father's round-crowned straw hat. The father sports an emphatically checked bow tie and tiny beard of the type popularized by Napoleon III.

96.
Little girl holding up her skirt to reveal a scalloped petticoat—a common and, undoubtedly, parent-pleasing photographer's ploy. Wrinkled stockings and ankle-strap shoes with bows.

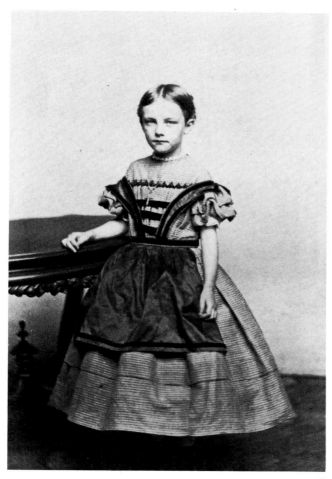

97

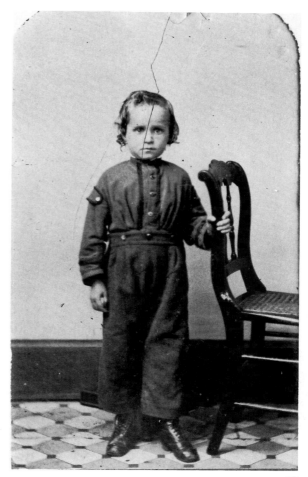

98

97.
"September 1863." Decorative aprons, never intended to see the inside of a kitchen, were
frequently worn by girls and women in the sixties
and early seventies.

98.
Boy in two-piece outfit with dark trim and
epaulets.

99.
Four boys in (left to right): Long pants with
matching vest and sack jacket; Garibaldi pants,
bolero jacket with contrasting trim, vest; suit with
peg-top trousers and applied decoration; skirt,
jacket, pantalets.

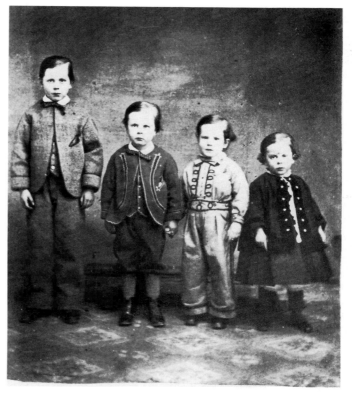

99

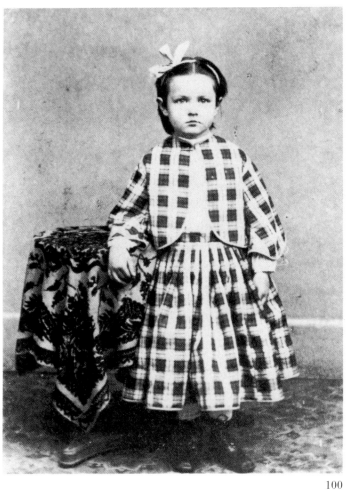

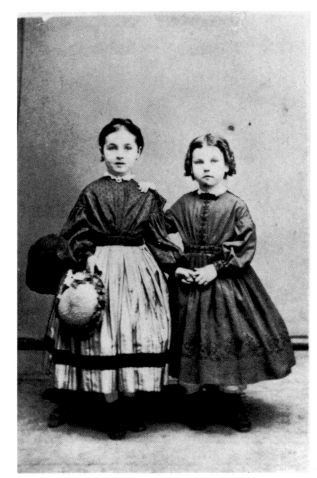

100

101

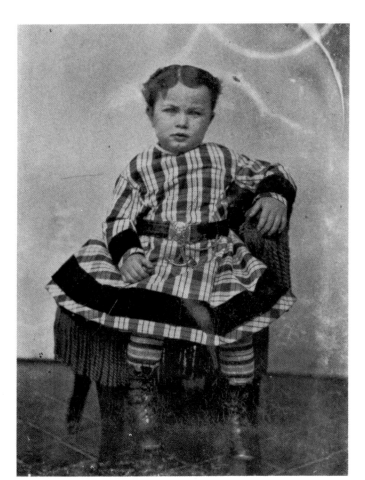

100.
Girl in matching tartan skirt and bolero jacket; hair ribbon.

101.
Sisters in "high Garibaldi" dresses (in reference to the neckline; "low Garibaldi" having a scoop neck) with very full sleeves, dropped shoulders and a band of trim near the hem.

102.
Boy in plaid dress with dark trim; a tiny hunting horn hangs from his belt; horizontally striped stockings.

102

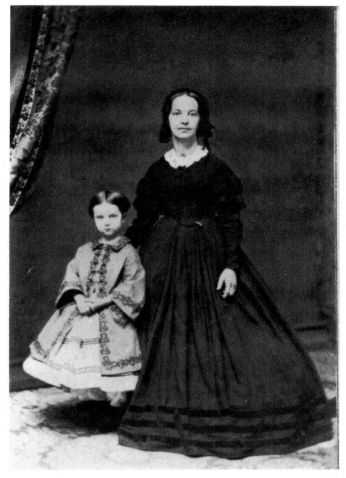

103

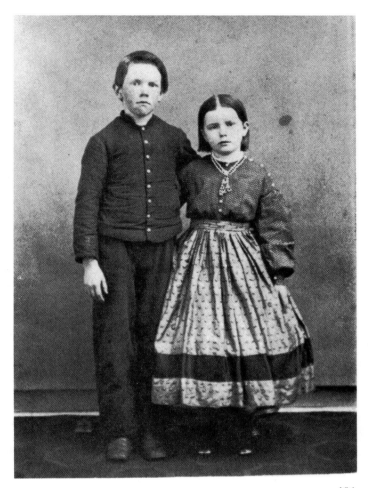

104

103.
"Mrs. —— Williams, Leavenworth, Kansas." Mother and daughter in hoopskirts. The little girl wears a three-quarter-length coat with flared sleeves and applied decoration.

104.
Boy in wrinkled straight-cut jacket that is almost outgrown; girl in a Garibaldi outfit—a dotted blouse and print skirt.

105.
Boy in round-cut jacket with slightly flared sleeves; long pants; military-style cap in hand.

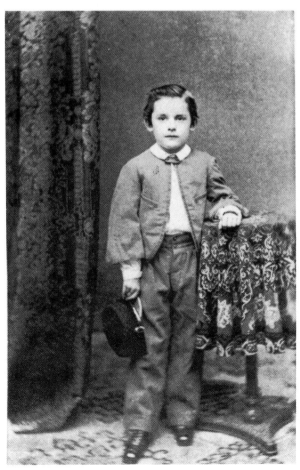

105

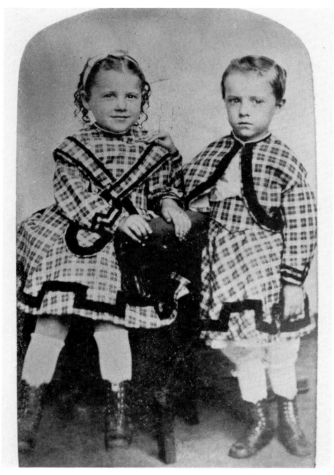

106

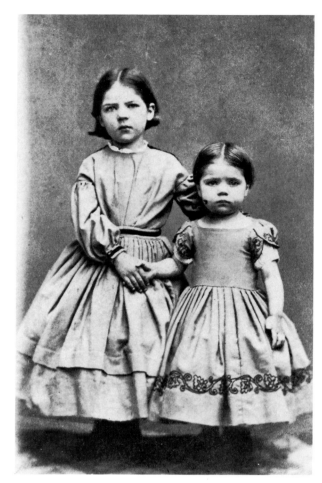

107

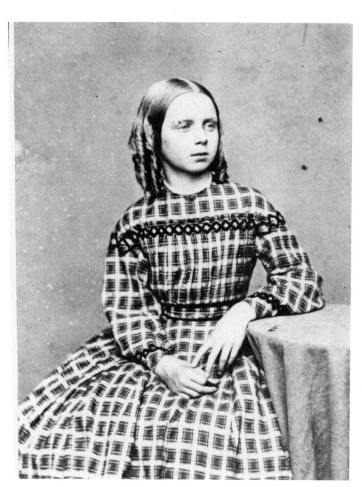

108

106.
Brother and sister in coordinated outfits of plaid with dark trim. She has wide bretelles; he has a bolero jacket.

107.
"Ida and Bertha," 1865. Ida's long sleeves are buttoned on; Bertha's skirt and tulip sleeves have applied decoration.

108.
Teenage girl in plaid dress with applied geometric trim. Corkscrew curls.

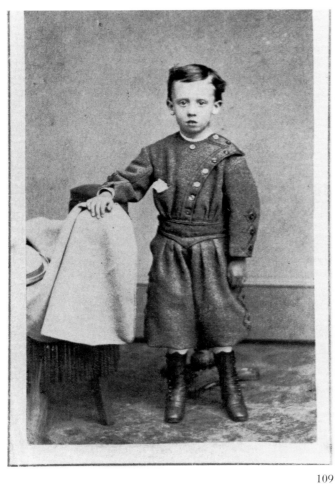

109

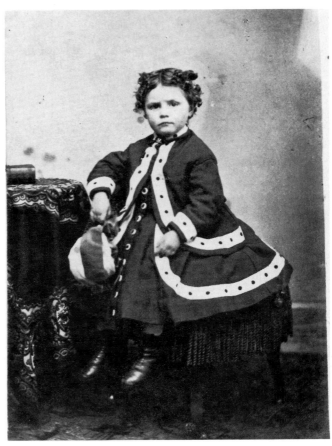

110

109.
Boy in suit with diagonally buttoned top; Garibaldi pants.

110.
Girl in dress with buttons down the front, white trim with black dots; matching short jacket; dated 1867.

111.
Boy in three-quarter-length checked pants; double-breasted coat with military-style cape and contrasting trim; dated 1867. (The subject is probably the brother of No. 110—the same photographer has used the same props.)

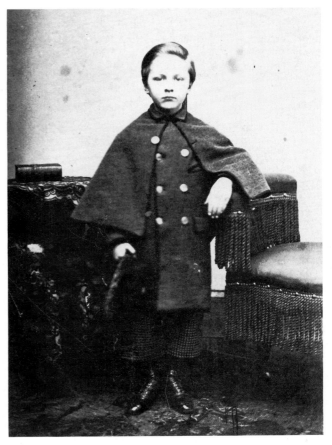

111

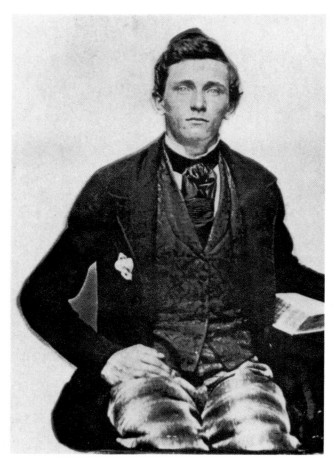

112

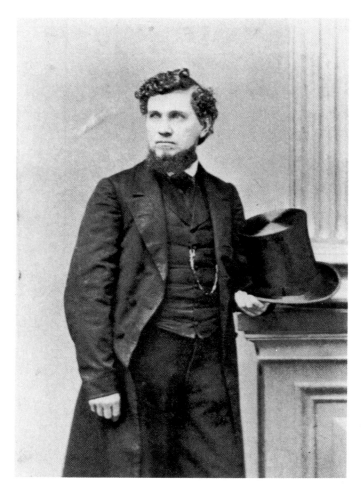

113

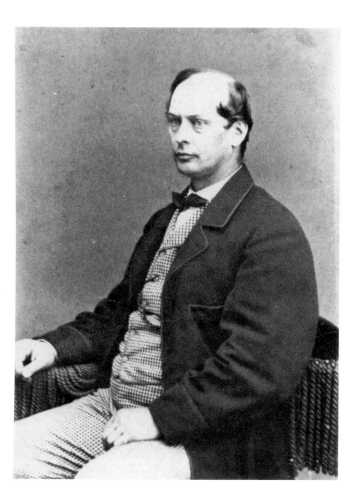

114

112.
Man in patterned trousers; shawl-collared brocaded waistcoat; wide made-up satin cravat.

113.
Bearded, curly haired gentleman in frock coat with matching vest; watch chain; top hat.

114.
"Chas. Douglas." The matching checked vest and trousers are very fashionable, as are the braid-trimmed sack coat and small bow tie.

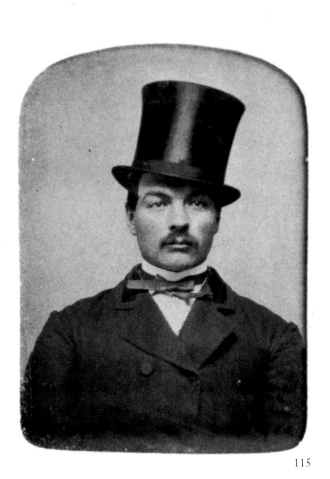

115

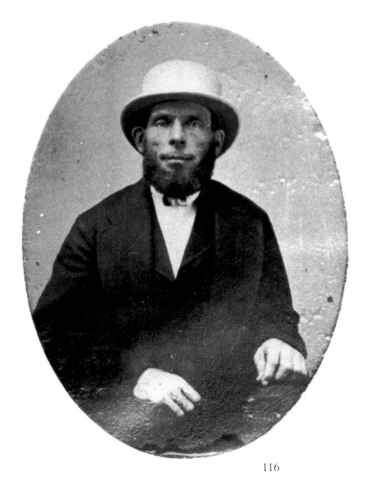

116

115.
Worn at a rakish angle, this man's top hat has slightly concave sides. The narrow standing collar was new in the sixties.

116.
The light-colored bowler apparently rests on the gentleman's ears.

117.
A very tall top hat, worn with the popular little bow tie; 1864–66.

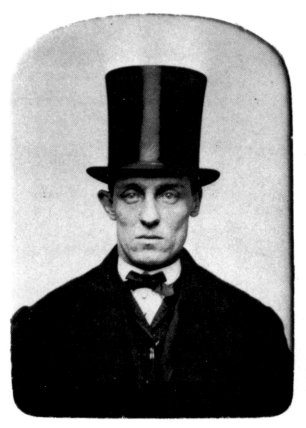

117

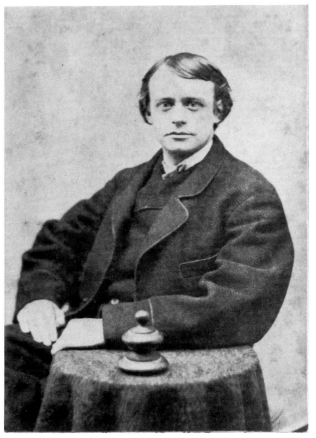

118

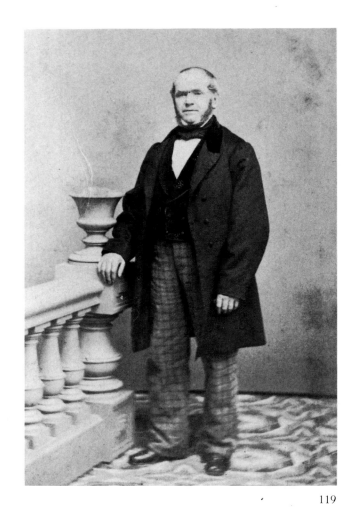

119

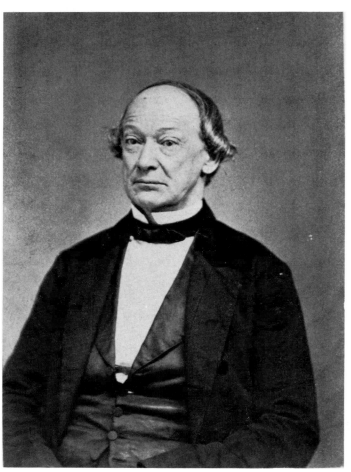

118.
Braid-trimmed wool sack coat with characteristic wide sleeves; matching vest; 1864–66.

119.
Bearded gentleman in double-breasted frock coat with velvet collar; shawl-collared, double-breasted vest; baggy plaid trousers.

120.
Older gentleman in low-standing collar still brushes his hair into a roll over the ears; satin vest.

120

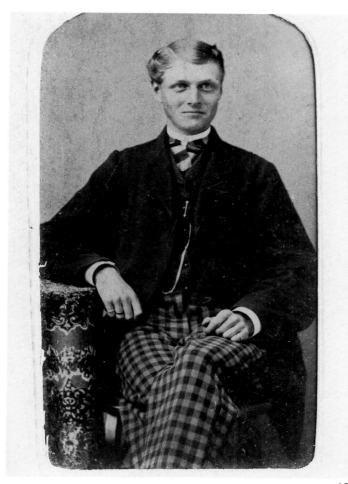

121

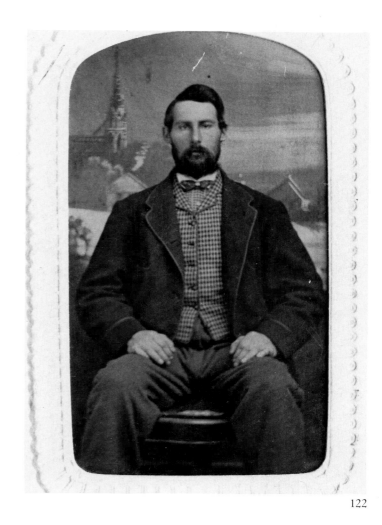

122

121.
This debonair man wears checked trousers with a dark coat, striped cravat and the new low round collar.

122.
Bearded man with solid-color unmatched coat and trousers; checked waistcoat; shirt in smaller check; white collar and small bow tie.

123.
Older man in tailcoat, top hat, rumpled trousers; cane; eyeglasses hang from his waistcoat.

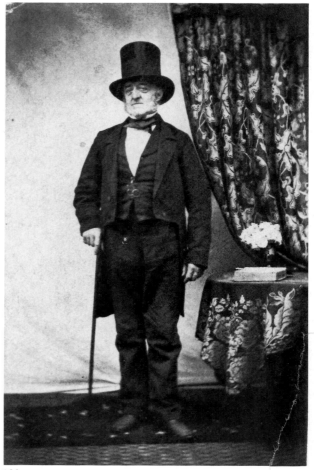

123

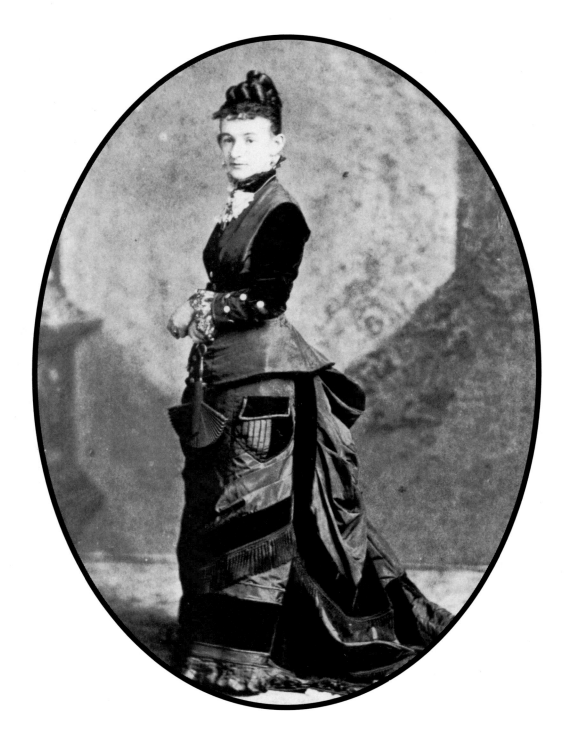

Modish gown, the ornamental pocket indicating
ca. 1876. See Figure 145.

The 1870s

The bustle quickly gained favor, growing by 1873 into a full-blown, short-waisted, bouffant style with draped overskirts, frequently a train, and embellished by seemingly endless combinations of such trimmings as pleats, bows, buttons, ruffles, chenille balls, ribbon and fringe. Wide sleeves made an occasional reappearance, though moderately narrow ones were more generally seen. Colors were apt to be vivid and rather harsh, now that aniline dyes, developed in the 1850s, were being used.

Hats and bonnets were still quite small. The latter, which now might be tied in the back instead of under the chin, continued to be de rigueur for more formal daytime occasions. Julia Grant complained that occasionally a lady would attend a noon White House reception without a bonnet, "which would indicate that she was one of the receiving party," but, she added rather ominously, "This little maneuver was never repeated by the same person."[1] There were times, of course, when a bonnet was *not* appropriate. An English visitor, attending a similar presidential reception held in the evening, reported in astonishment that one " 'lady' . . . scorning the cloak-room, where perhaps, she feared her outer garments would get pilfered or exchanged, walked in with her bonnet and waterproof, an umbrella in her hand, and her overshoes under her arm."[2]

Women's hair might simply be pulled back into a snood, or piled up into a chignon, perhaps topped by plump braids. It could also be worn loose, shoulder-length or longer, and a "fringe" of curly bangs was increasingly seen. Fringed cravat bows or lacy jabots were worn at the throat, and velvet neck ribbons, heavy gold-chain or jet necklaces, crosses, gold bracelets, pendant earrings and other jewelry were common. Fans and elaborate parasols completed the costume. The overall look was fussy, and just a hairsbreadth away from being frowsy.

By the mid-seventies the bustle had begun to diminish, its fullness moving lower and lower and gradually becoming more restrained. A tightly fitting, boned, long-waisted bodice, known as a basque bodice (or cuirass basque), which extended over the hips, smoothed out the upper portion of the gown. There was a great deal of interest in asymmetrical effects. The skirt, though narrower, continued to be draped and gathered, and was almost always trained, even for daytime wear.

The prevalence of such trains throughout the decade posed some special problems. "The woman cannot be self-respecting who can trail a long skirt across a muddy street, entailing not only the ruin of the dress, but the certain bedaubing of stockings and underclothes . . . ," wrote Ethel Gale, adding, "that there are many women thus unfortunately devoid of self-respect, the daily scenes in our streets assure us."[3] A partial solution was the inexpensive dust ruffle or "balayeuse." Sewn onto the underside of the train, it could easily be ripped out and washed when soiled, or simply thrown away and replaced. Nevertheless, the train of even the most fastidious woman must have been, on occasion, a rather sorry and bedraggled sight.

The trend toward a slimmer line continued, and by the late seventies the princess dress, its form-fitting line unbroken by any waist seams, was also in vogue. What drapery there was occurred below the hips at the back of the skirt, which was now so small in circumference that it had a hobbling effect. The bustle had been temporarily vanquished. Hats grew somewhat higher in the crown and were more heavily decorated.

For men, the sack coat and the suit, with matched components, were increasingly seen for casual wear, worn with bowlers, and, in the summer, low-crowned straw hats. There was a new emphasis on textured materials, and lapels were cut wider and longer. The frock coat and top hat were still necessary for more formal occasions. Double-breasted Chesterfields with velvet collars were popular overcoats. Beards were shorter, and there were more mustaches. Hair was worn fairly short and was no longer brushed forward to curl over the ears. A few fashionable young men challenged tradition and appeared with a center part. This was not well received by the average American, whose reaction was said to be typified by General Grant, "who disliked on sight any man whose hair was parted in the middle."[4]

Girls wore ruffles and overskirts and, occasionally, a big bow at the back of the waist. Decorative aprons were fashionable. Girls' hair might be shoulder-length, sometimes with bangs, but most continued to wear it in the simple styles of the sixties. Although small boys still wore dresses or kilts, the fashion for off-shoulder dresses and pantalets for both sexes was at last on the wane. Boys, when breeched, were now seldom put directly into long pants; instead they wore knickers, or other below-the-knee pants, with side-buttoned tunics or various jackets. The hair was worn quite short. Checks and plaids were popular for all children, as were horizontally striped stockings and boots. For work or vigorous play, girls wore simple and comfortable dresses, and boys wore collarless shirts with low-set full sleeves, plain pants and suspenders.

---

[1] Grant, *op. cit.*, p. 176.
[2] *Our American Cousins at Home*, Vera (London: Sampson Low, Marston, Low and Searle, 1873), p. 193.
[3] *Hints on Dress*, Ethel Gale (New York: Putnam, 1872), p. 27.
[4] *Mornings on Horseback*, David McCullough (New York: Simon & Schuster, 1981), p. 203.

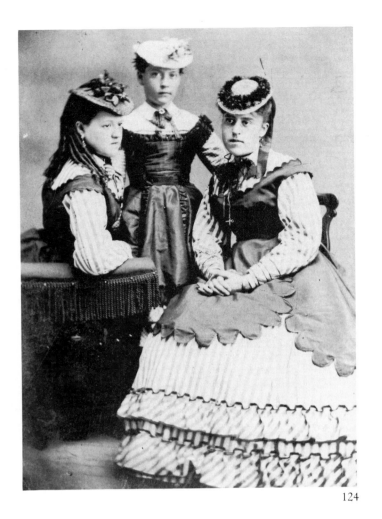

124

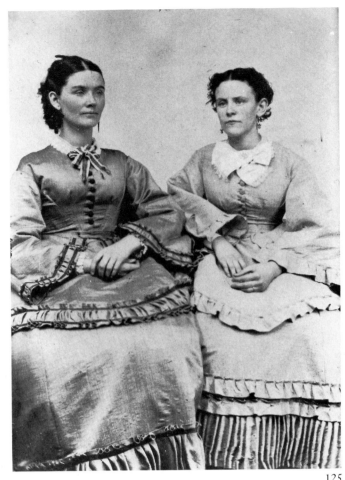

125

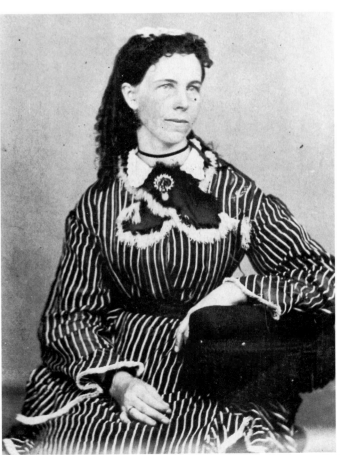

126

124.
Decorative apron-effect dresses on three young women. Two wear identical striped dresses; all have tiny flat-crowned hats tilted over the forehead. Note the long, shiny curls of the girl on left and the miniature scissors worn on a cord by girl on right.

125.
Wide sleeves were popular in 1870. Here they are worn by two women in gowns with overskirts; pleats and gathers; tight bodices; neck bows.

126.
Lady in vividly striped dress; fringed scarf; long curls.

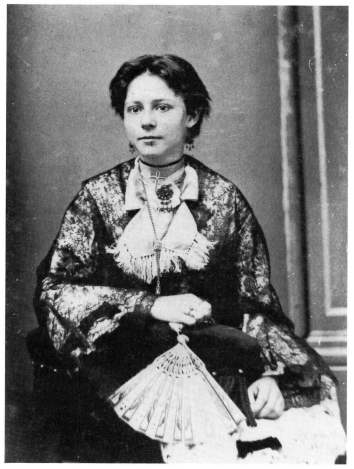

127

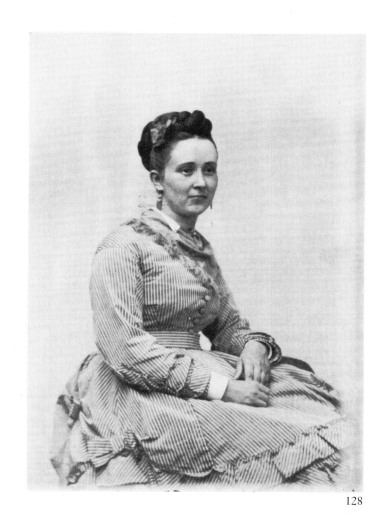

128

127.
Lady with short-cropped hair (perhaps the result of illness), but in all other respects typifying the early seventies with her Chantilly lace jacket; velvet neck ribbon with cross; matching brooch and pendant earrings; large fringed neck bow; necklace; fan.

128.
Overskirt with back fullness; fringe, bows, ruffles and stripes (stripes being particularly smart in the late sixties and early seventies).

129.
Curly bangs, striped dress with bustle; lacy collar, cuffs and jabot; necklace and brooch.

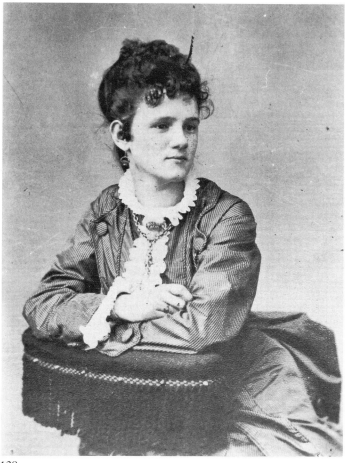

129

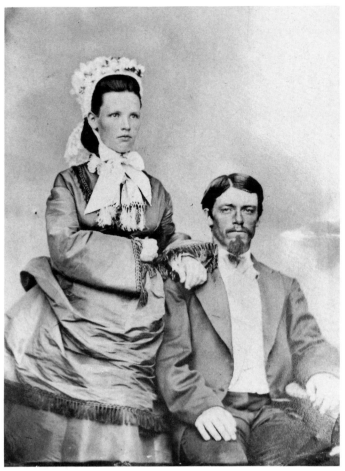

130

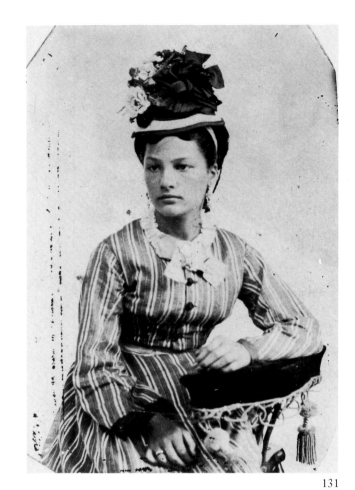

131

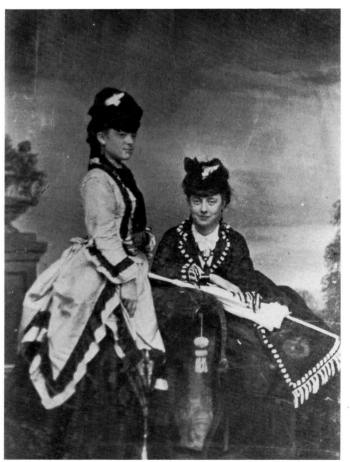

132

130.
The woman's small, flower-covered bonnet is set well back on the head; the "strings" now pass behind the ears to tie under the chin in a large bow that almost obscures the fringed jabot underneath; gown with overskirt trimmed with fringe, as are the cuffs and bodice. The man's rather wide-sleeved coat has the new, longer lapels.

131.
A bonnet with ribbons and bows ties in back of this young woman's chignon.

132.
The "Dolly Varden" polonaise (left), a gathered-up overskirt with its roots in the eighteenth century (but taking its name from a character in Dickens' *Barnaby Rudge*), was a passing fad in the early seventies. Small hats; parasols.

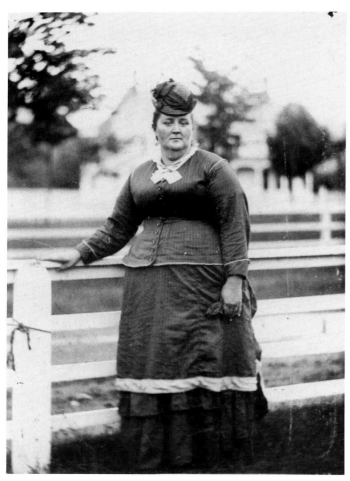

133

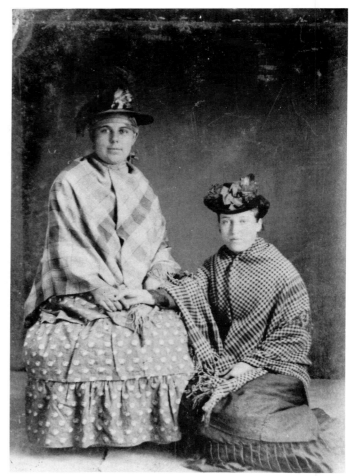

134

133.
Women of little means adapted current fashions to fit their purse. Here a tight bodice is worn with a poorly made overskirt, with some back draping just visible. Tiny hat tilted forward.

134.
Shawls, the most economical type of outer garment, could be pinned together to leave the arms free.

135.
Teenage girls in simple dresses with belted overskirts. Age still determines length of skirt. A fan hangs from belt of girl on right.

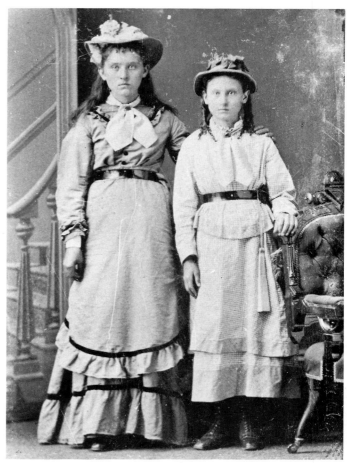

135

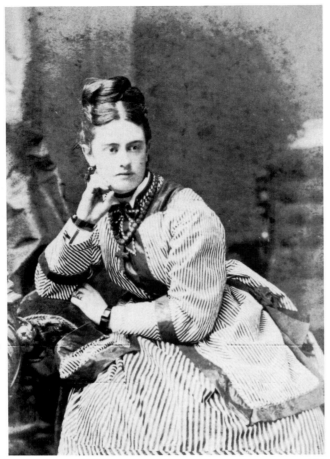

136

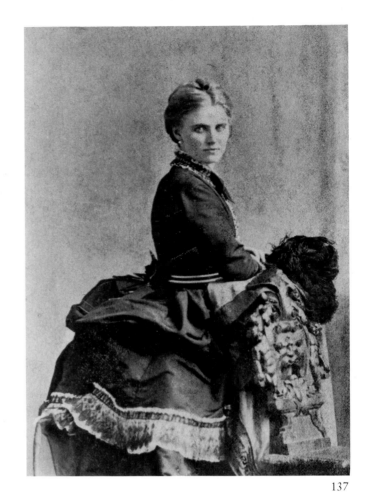

137

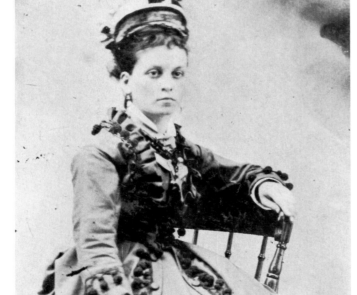

138

136.
Lady in boldly striped skirt with tunic in finer stripe and dark trim; bustle; cross, bracelets; hair in large braid.

137.
Gown with short-waisted, belted bodice and full bustle; overskirt trimmed with wide embroidered band.

138.
Chenille-ball fringe trim, in addition to ruffles, decorate this bustled polonaise, which opens in front to reveal an underskirt with successive bands of tucks and pleats.

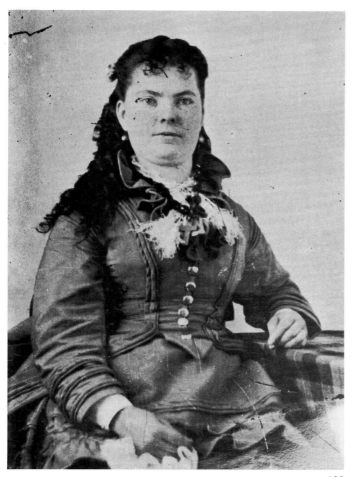

139

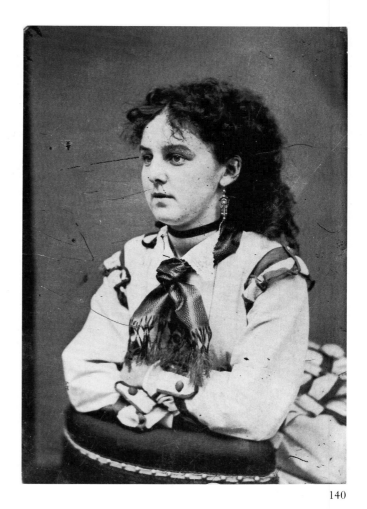

140

139.
Lady with short basque bodice, ruffles, fringe, cross, long curls and handkerchief.

140.
Long hair, curly bangs, pendant earrings, velvet neck ribbon, fringed and knotted scarf and a ruffled bustle.

141.
The woman wears the seventies bustle seen in full flower, complete with train. The gentleman wears a suit with wide, long lapels; his trousers flare out at the bottom.

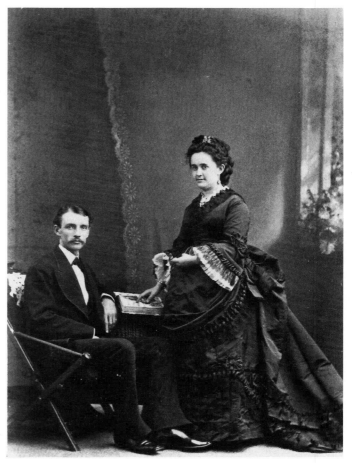

141

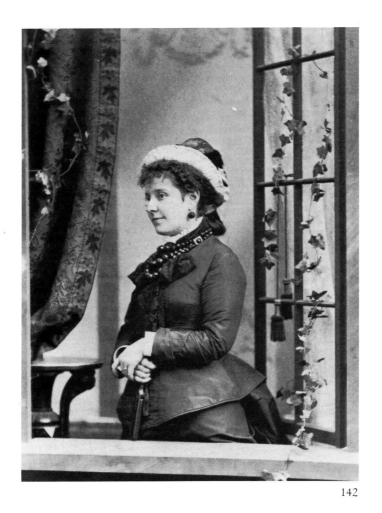

142

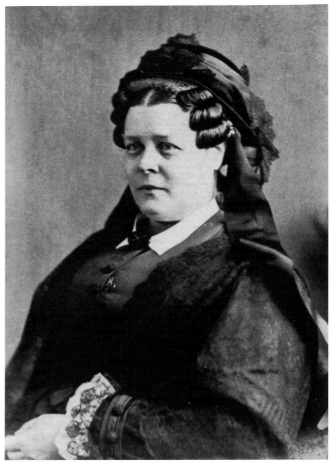

143

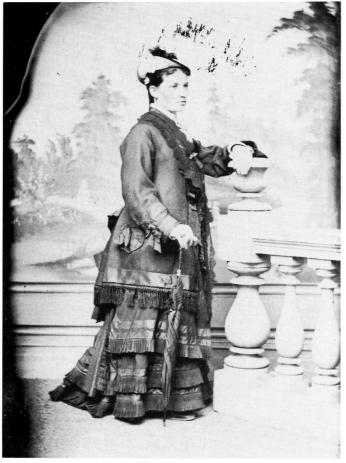

144

142.
An early version of the basque bodice, pointed in front, with the shorter back jutting out over the bustle. Heavy jewelry like this triple-strand necklace with matching earrings was in vogue.

143.
A matron in a small hat with broad ribbons, and what are almost certainly false curls. Many women were reluctant to cut their long hair and resorted to hair pieces to create the desired fashionable effects.

144.
In the mid-seventies skirts became narrower and the rear draping was lower and more restrained. This stylish outfit, with its matching hip-length coat, includes the decorative pocket that was fashionable in 1875 and 1876. Train; umbrella.

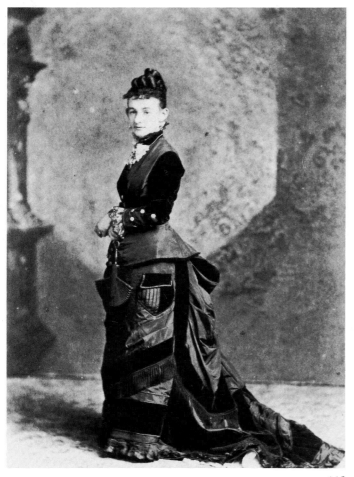

145

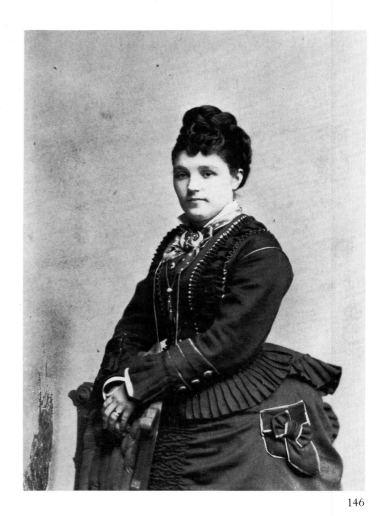

146

145.
A modish gown trimmed with fringe, ruffles and bands of dark velvet; decorative pocket; long basque bodice; fan; dust ruffle visible under train. The glistening curls are probably not the lady's own.

146.
The external decorative pocket dates this gown from 1875–76, although the bodice is shorter and the bustle higher and more pronounced than usually seen.

147.
Two fashionable ladies. Several layers of knife pleats decorate the hemline at the left; on the right, pleats and ruching, which borders the overskirt; trains; umbrella.

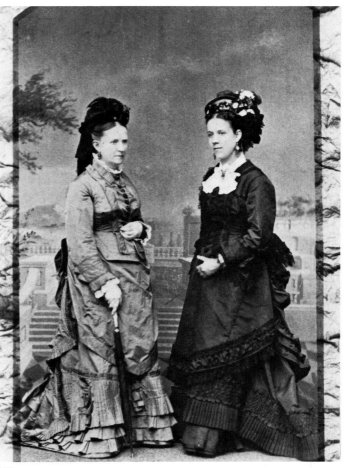

147

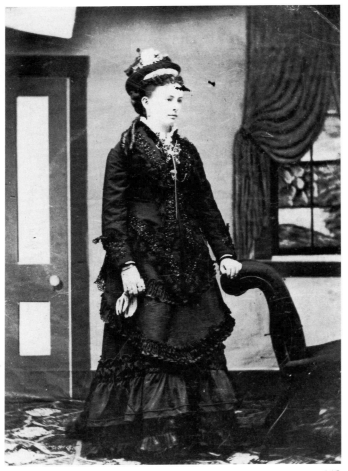

148

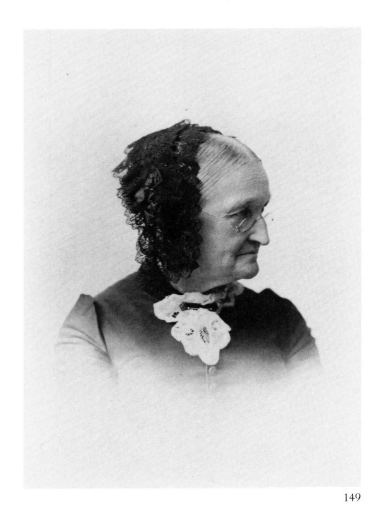

149

148.
Jet-trimmed bodice; double pointed overskirts with ruched trim; underskirt with deep flounce; two long curls over shoulder; small hat on top of head; gloves in hand.

149.
Older lady in black Chantilly lace house cap; spectacles. Only the elderly still wore caps indoors.

150.
Velvet trim was very popular in the mid-seventies; here it decorates the bodice, overskirt and bustle. Underskirt with three flounces of knife pleats.

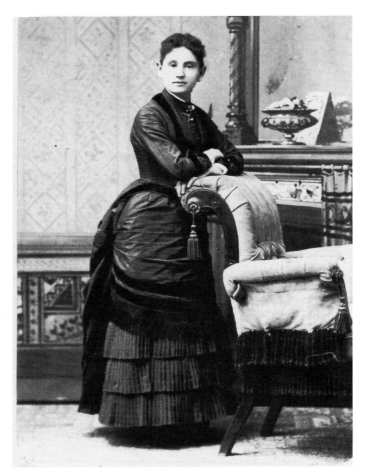

150

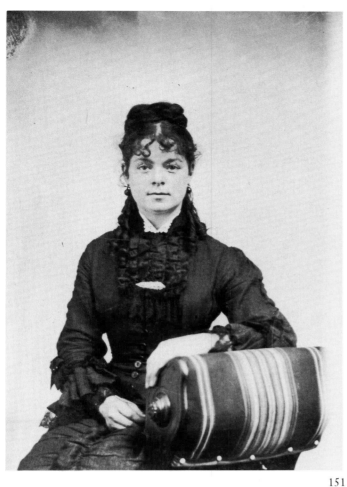

151

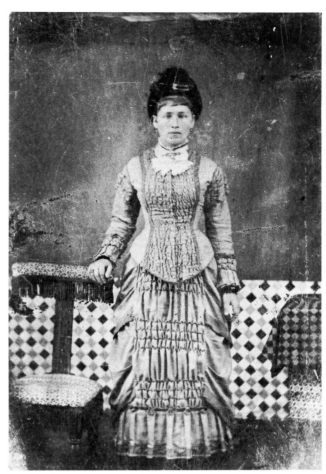

152

151.
Young woman in princess dress with satin jabot and pleated and lacy cuffs. A slimmer look prevailed in the late seventies.

152.
As the eighties approached, shirring was very fashionable, and is used here in wide panels on both the skirt and the basque bodice.

153.
The man wears a checked coat, lighter checked trousers and a cap. The woman is in a dress with ruching on the bodice, sleeves and overskirt; the underskirt has knife pleats and ruffle.

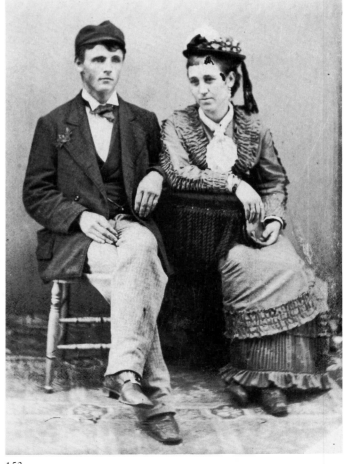

153

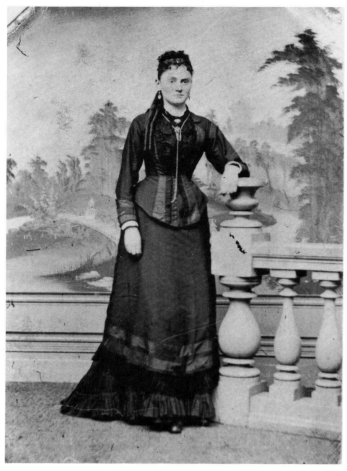

154

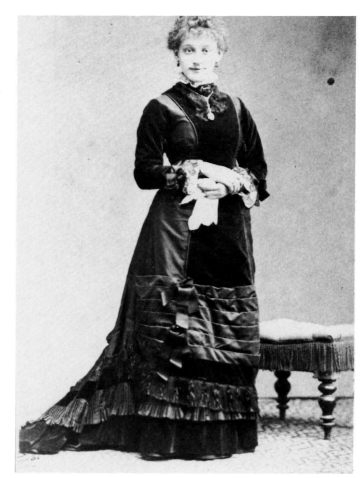

155

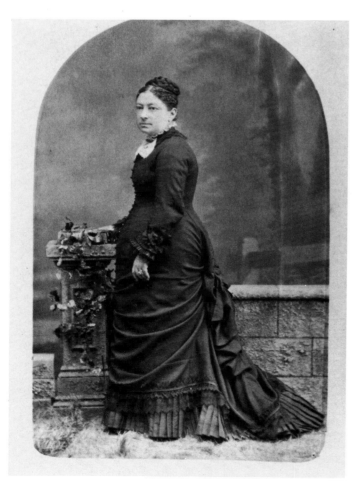

156

154.
Excellent example of the "armored effect" of the late seventies basque (or cuirass) bodice, boned and extremely form-fitting. The line now is long and slender.

155.
"Carrie Gilmore." Trained satin-and-velvet gown with pleats, bows and rows of tucks; frilly cuffs and collar; dark lace jabot; necklace; handkerchief.

156.
Lady in princess dress with train.

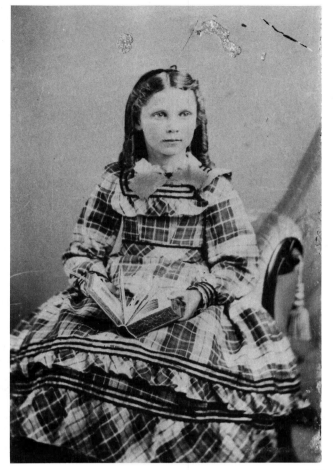

157

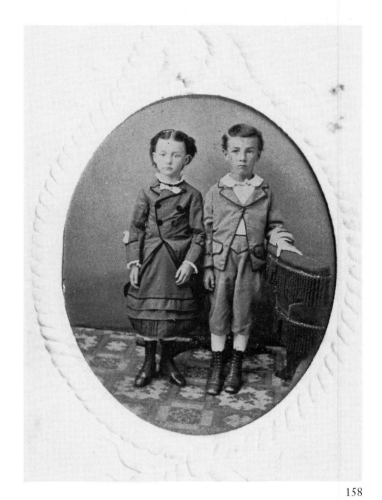

158

157.
"Lunette Augusta Fuller Hallett." The girl, with long curls, wears a plaid dress with ruffled overskirt; bodice with square ruffle-edged yoke.

158.
Girl and boy in similarly trimmed outfits. She is in a double-breasted cutaway coat over a skirt with two rows of tucks and a pleated hem. He wears calf-length pants and a top-buttoned jacket.

159.
"Willie C. Winks, May 7, 1870, ACB." Off-shoulder dress with pleated bodice, ribbons at shoulders, scalloped hem and braid trim.

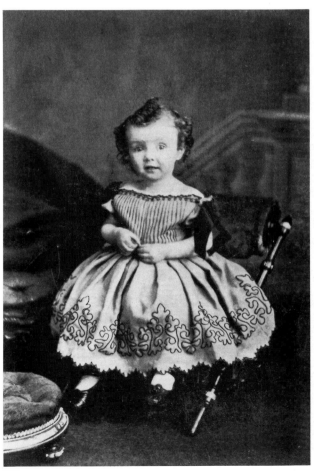

159

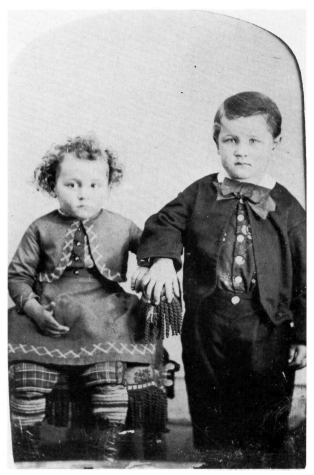

160

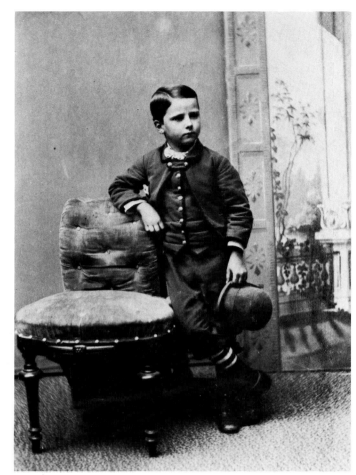

161

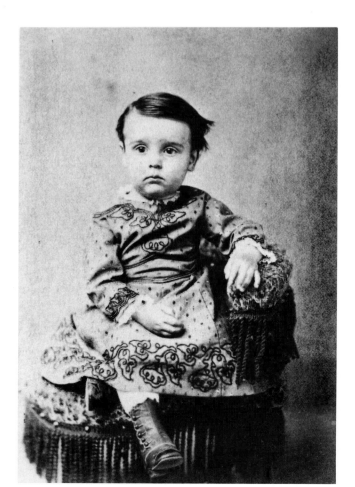

162

160.
The younger boy is in a bolero jacket and matching skirt over checked pants and horizontally striped stockings; the older is in an unusual floral print blouse that must have been made from the remnants of a female relative's dress. It buttons to the pants and is worn with a short, drop-shouldered jacket and big bow tie.

161.
Boy with three-quarter-length pants, jacket with tab closing, and vest—all braid-trimmed; striped stockings; high-crowned hat.

162.
Little boy in diamond-patterned dress with elaborate soutache trim at hem, neckline and cuffs.

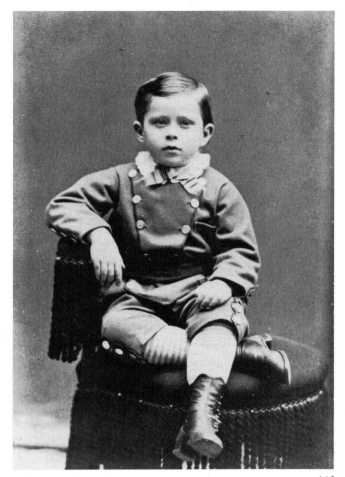

163

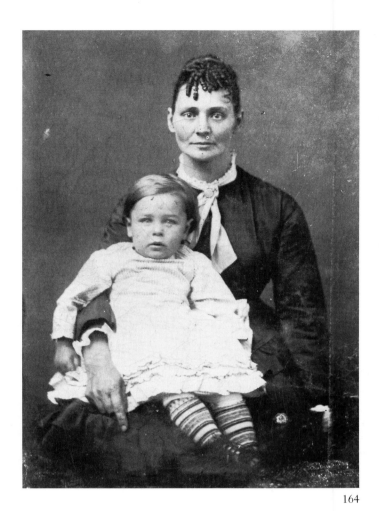

164

163.
Buttons trim the pants, sleeves and front of this boy's outfit.

164.
Boy in ruffled dress and striped stockings; his mother has a cluster of tiny corkscrew curls on her forehead.

165.
Boy in two-piece wool sailor-style outfit trimmed with bands of white; separate collar, striped stockings, high-button shoes.

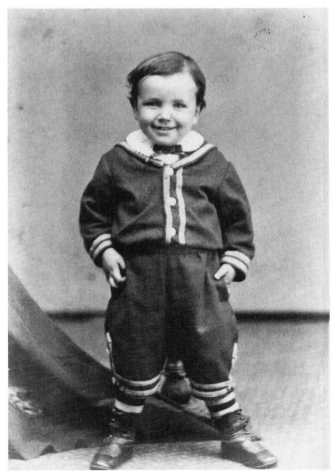

165

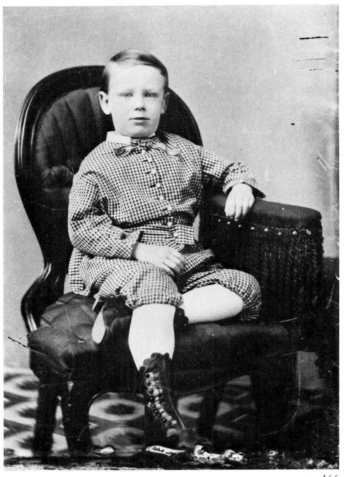

166

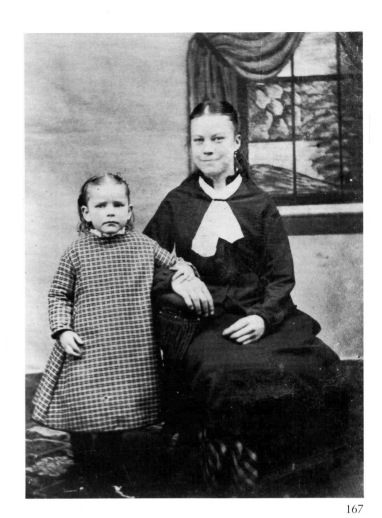

167

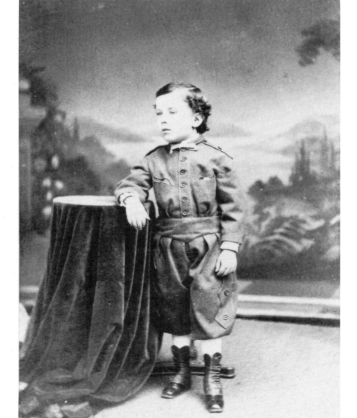

168

166.
Boy in checked belted tunic with matching knickerbockers.

167.
The little girl is in an absolutely plain long-sleeved, checked dress.

168.
"George Probasco or little *Pod* for short." Little boy in two-piece wool suit with button trim.

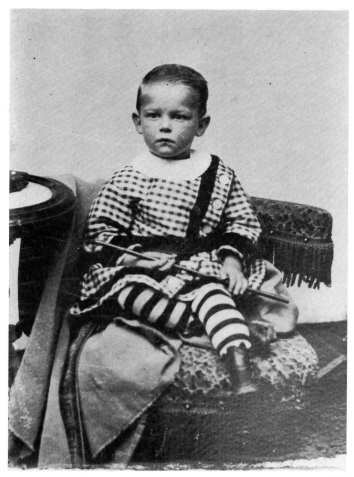

169

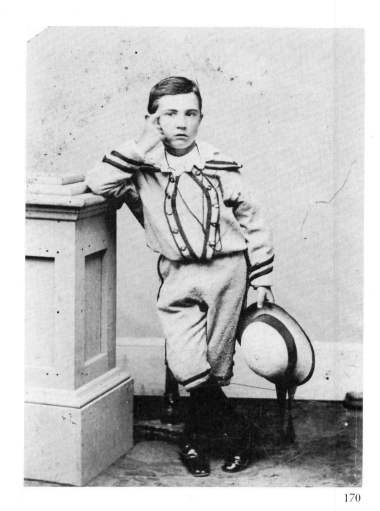

170

169.
Little boy in checked, side-buttoned dress with dark trim; white collar, striped stockings. He holds a cane.

170.
Boy holding straw hat with ribbons. He wears a two-piece suit decorated with buttons and bands of dark trim.

171.
Little girl in a flounced, ruffled skirt, with more ruffles at cuffs and on bodice; buttoned boots.

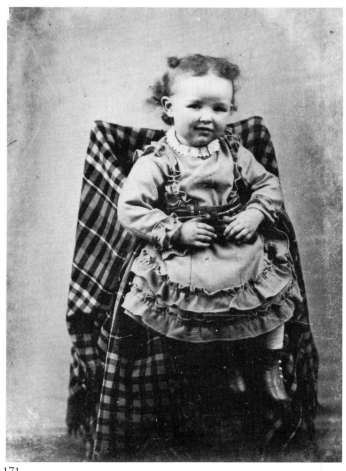

171

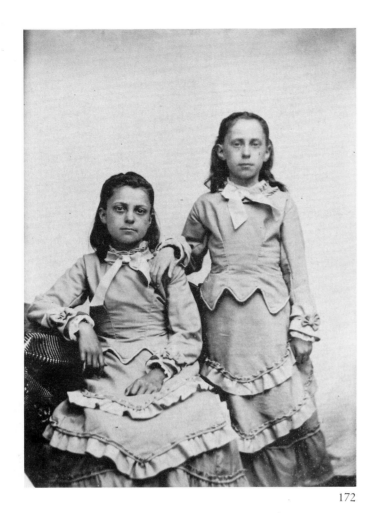

172

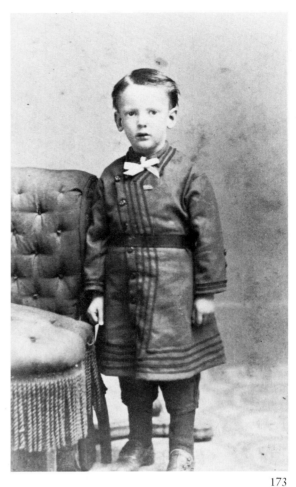

173

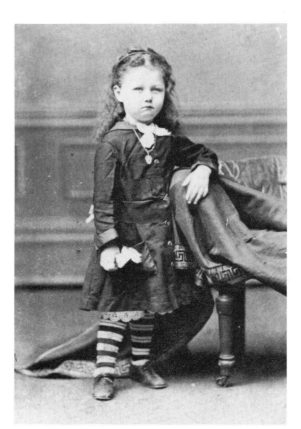

174

172.
Sisters in identical dresses with tri-pointed bodice, pointed and ruffle-trimmed overskirts, darker underskirt, bows on cuffs; long hair.

173.
Boy in side-buttoned, belted tunic trimmed with four rows of braid; tight pants that stop above the ankle; dark stockings.

174.
"Hattie Smith." Long hair and hair ribbon; dress with exterior pocket; striped stockings.

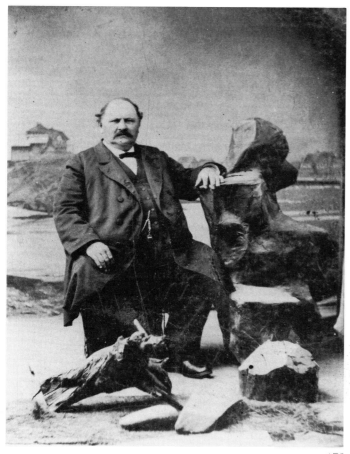

175

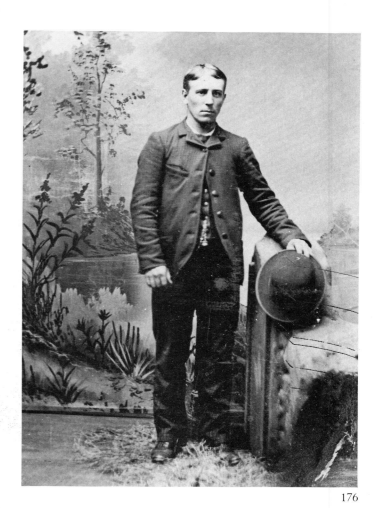

176

175.
Gentleman in frock coat and narrow bow tie.

176.
High-buttoned sack coat; round-crowned hat; short hair.

177.
Bearded gentleman in the somewhat lower top hat of the seventies; sack coat.

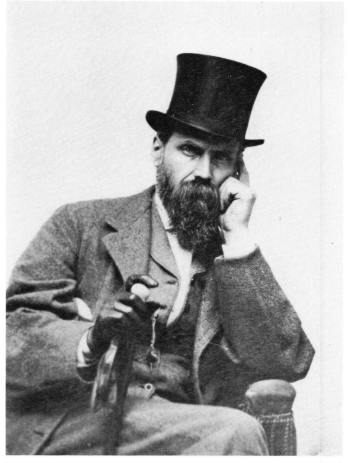

177

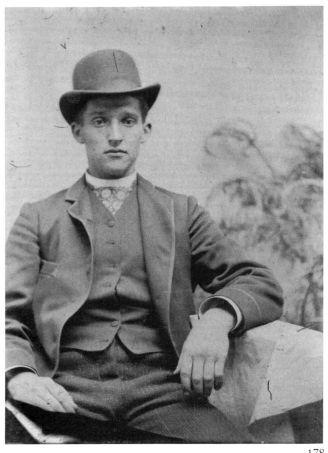

178

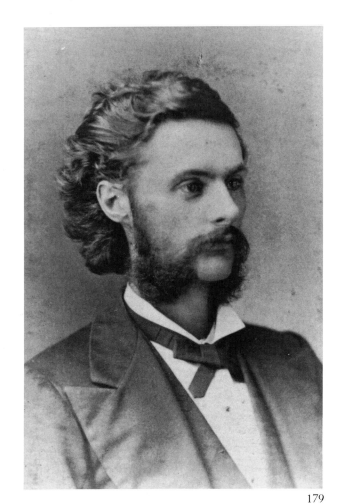

179

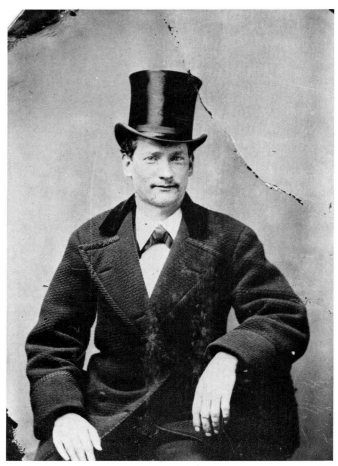

180

178.
Curving-brimmed bowler, worn with matching sack coat and vest, odd trousers, low round collar and wide, patterned necktie.

179.
"Louis De Lamartor Nov 20, 1876." Wing collar, small bow tie, wide lapels, long wavy hair brushed away from face.

180.
Braid-trimmed, double-breasted Chesterfield of heavy textured material with wide lapels; top hat.

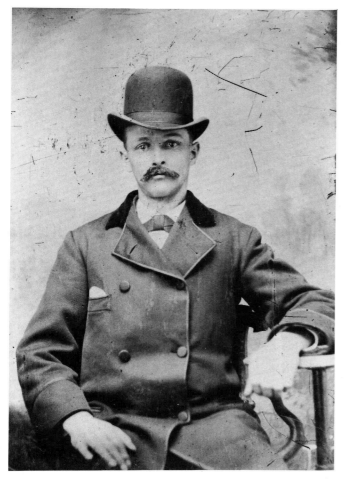

181

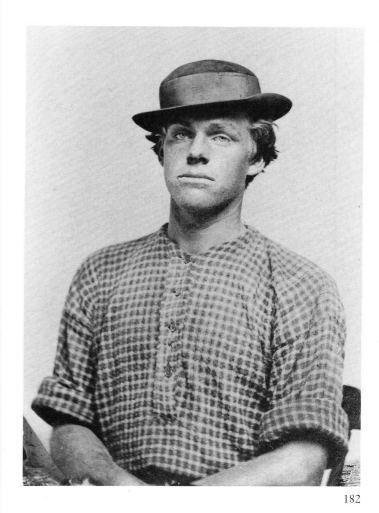

182

181.
Gentleman in high-crowned, curving-brimmed bowler; double-breasted overcoat; turned-down collar and small bow tie.

182.
Man in a typical nineteenth-century workshirt of collarless checked flannel with four-button opening (or placket); low-crowned derby.

183.
Bearded man with cap and earrings. His matching coat and double-breasted, shawl-collared vest are of a small-checked material.

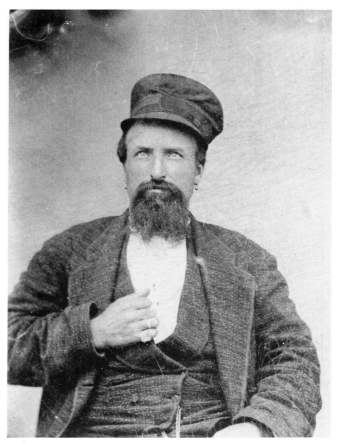

183

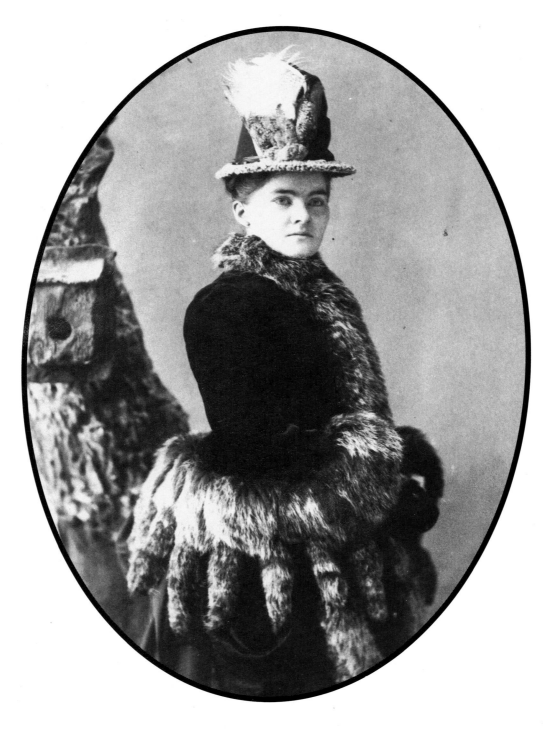

"Kate Lears, 1885." See Figure 204.

The 1880s

The slim look of the late seventies continued briefly. Narrow skirts and high necks were countered by extremely fitted basque bodices, tiny waists and trim hiplines that revealed the rigidly corseted torso with new distinctness. Only the princess dress and the polonaise (a long, coatlike bodice drawn up in folds over the skirt) offered some slight relief from the tightly sheathed look. That the latter did not please everyone is evident from a letter Woodrow Wilson wrote to his fiancée, Ellen Axson, in 1885, concerning her trousseau preparations. He urged her to avoid close-fitting basque bodices that give "a rigid, stayed appearance . . . . A basque form that goes below the waist and is reinforced with whalebones, or the like, is terrible to look upon . . . real beauty [is in] bodices which suggest, rather than outline the figure . . . ."[1]

Trains were now almost never seen during the day, except in tea gowns worn strictly at home. There was a good deal of intricate draping and trimming of the skirt and overskirt, and renewed interest in asymmetrical effects. Sleeves often were not full length, stopping anywhere below the elbow. The back of the skirt, below the hips, remained the focal point at first, but, by 1882, had risen once again into a new version of the bustle. With the line of the dress in front quite straight (thanks to the use of interior tapes to tie it back), this current and very emphatic protuberance produced a startling effect. It had none of the billowing softness of its predecessor in the seventies, but, by the mid-eighties, in its most extreme form, it jutted out at a right angle to the back. It is no wonder that visitors from the East sometimes asked if Western women were physically deformed.

It is hard to reconcile this bizarre style with a social climate that produced a reference to "the young woman of today, . . . skating, driving and bicycling, studying chemistry in the laboratory, exhibiting pictures in open competition, adopting a profession without opposition, and living single without fear of reproach . . . ."[2] It is equally difficult to picture ladies playing tennis in their long skirts, with or without a bustle, but snapshots (the amateur camera having come on the scene in 1888) prove they did. What's more, some of them leaped over the net when the game was over!

The preoccupation with asymmetry eventually extended to the bodice, where a completely different material, often handled in a different way, might crop up on one side, with very little apparent relation to anything else in the dress. There was also the use of heavy fabrics, more than one textile in the same color, and what can be called the "upholstery effect." The result was unusual, to say the least. By this time the bustle was again beginning to subside, and a hint of fullness at the shoulders indicated the direction fashion was to take in the following decade.

Hair was worn up, generally with some soft fullness and curly or frizzy bangs. Unique to the eighties was a fondness for a fringe of elaborate spit curls across the forehead, sometimes looped through narrow ribbons attached to the hat. Hats themselves were moderate in size, generally with high crowns, and one fashionable new style looked exactly like an inverted flowerpot. Decoration could include flowers, berries, feathers, plumes, birds' wings and even the entire stuffed bird. Parasols, fans and umbrellas were common accessories.

Of men's fashions, one Isaac Walker said four styles were here to stay: the sack coat, the frock coat, the four-button cutaway and the dress coat. The comfortable sack coat was appropriate "except where extreme dignity is required," but "the nattiest garment that has come into vogue in recent years" was the four-button cutaway. It showed off a good figure perfectly, while the double-breasted frock coat "suffers because of the rectangular aspect and the superabundance of cloth."[3] Except for the evening dress coat, they almost always buttoned high at the neck, lapels were small and the fit on the tight side. Trousers might be checked or solid, and usually did not match the coat, except in the lounge suit. Since collars of coats buttoned so high, the high, tight collar predominated on shirts, with a narrow bow tie. Bowlers, boaters and caps were worn, as well as the top hat when the occasion demanded it. It was now becoming less unusual to see a man with a center part, although the side part still prevailed.

Little boys had not yet escaped from dresses. An 1880 pattern book shows 19 styles suitable for boys ages one to six, two to seven, and three to eight. For boys and girls, dresses tended to be straight and low-waisted, many with various combinations of pleats, scallops, ruffles and shirring. Most of this was concentrated on the lower third of the outfit, and there was sometimes a large bow at the rear. Lace collars were almost universal. Striped stockings were still seen. Bangs for the girls were common.

For parties and special events, boys had to endure what we now call the Little Lord Fauntleroy look—a velvet jacket or vest, with matching skirt or knee pants, a blouse with an extremely wide lace collar and lace cuffs, often a big sash at the waist, and, if possible, long curly hair. Knee pants now might be worn up to the age of 12, when long pants could be postponed no longer. Older boys and girls wore clothes similar to their elders. Butterick's pattern books in 1882 and 1885 show a number of "misses' dresses" for ages eight to 15 that look exactly like the current women's styles.

---

[1] *The Priceless Gift*, Ellen Wilson McAdoo (New York: McGraw-Hill, 1962), p. 136.

[2] *Louisa May Alcott*, Ednah D. Cheney (reprint of 1889 edition, New York: Chelsea House, 1981), p. 59.

[3] *Dress: As It Has Been, Is, and Will Be*, Isaac Walker (New York: published by the author, 1885), p. 119.

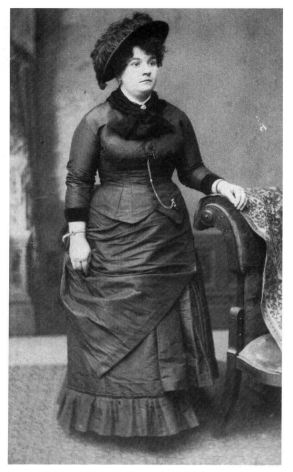

184

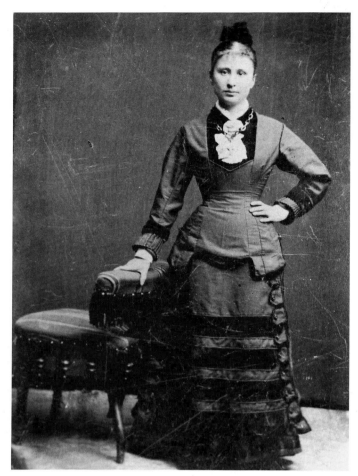

185

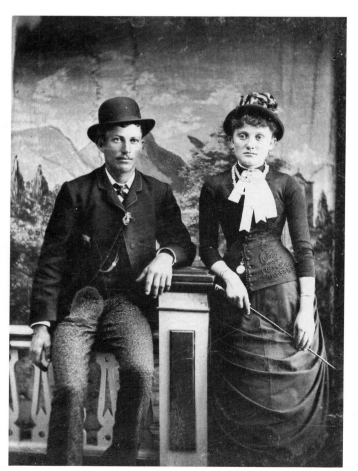

186

184.
Lady in basque bodice, asymmetrically draped and pleated overskirt, large plumed hat worn at an angle.

185.
Exceptionally long basque bodice trimmed with velvet as is the slim skirt with its decorative buttoned tabs on the sides.

186.
The man wears finely checked trousers and a high-buttoned sack coat and bowler. The woman displays a pocket watch on a sleek basque bodice decorated with applied trim; tight, three-quarter sleeves; draped overskirt.

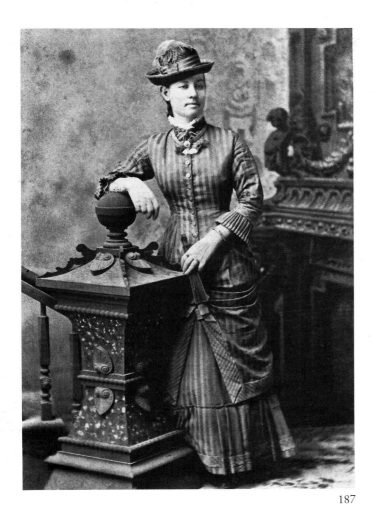

187

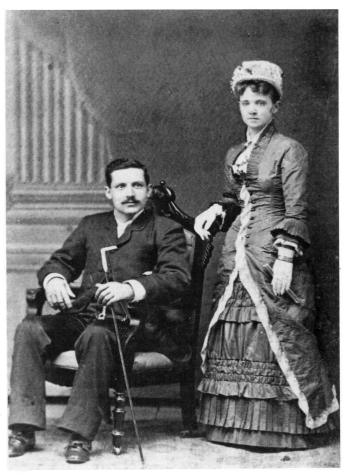

188

187.
Lady wearing a striped polonaise trimmed in a finer stripe used on the bias; gloves; fan; hat forward on brow.

188.
The woman offers another excellent example of the polonaise, here trimmed with white and worn with an underskirt having ruffles, shirring and pleats. The man is in a top-buttoned coat and holds a walking stick.

189.
Sisters frequently dressed alike, even when grown up. These two wear very tight basque bodices with diagonally applied decoration; unpressed-pleated skirts. (The photographer's head clamp is visible at left.) The gentleman wears a three-piece suit and narrow bow tie and holds a bowler.

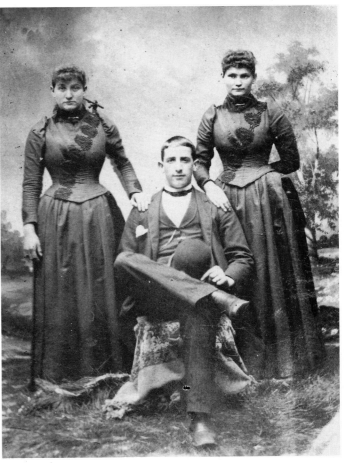

189

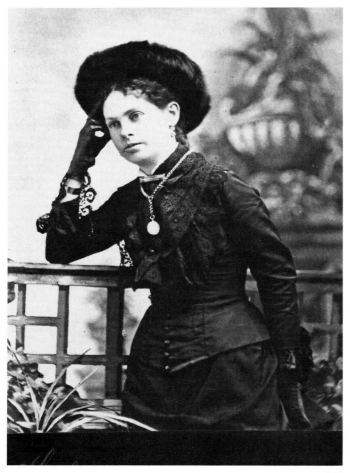

190

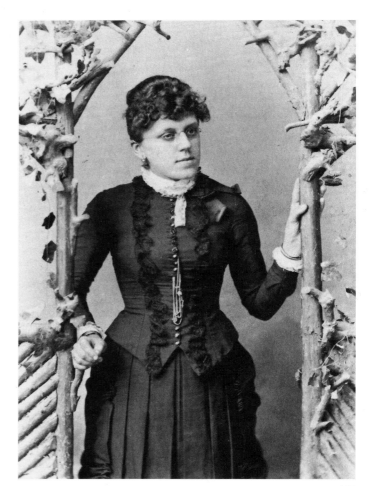

191

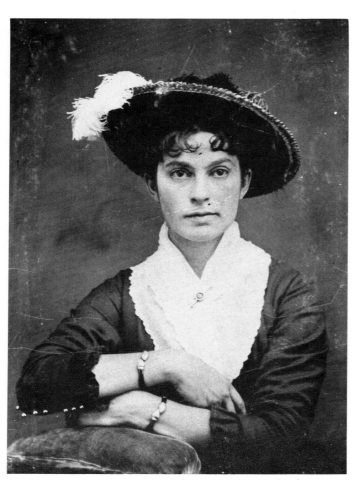

192

190.
Lady with black lace at cuffs and as a fichu; necklace with locket; gloves; fur hat.

191.
Lady wearing a basque bodice with lace trim; pleated skirt.

192.
Young woman with three-quarter sleeves, identical bracelets on each wrist, white fichu, curly bangs and wide-brimmed hat with plume.

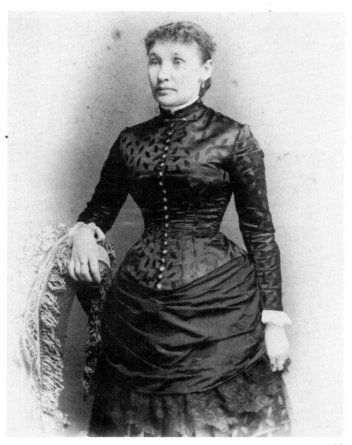

193

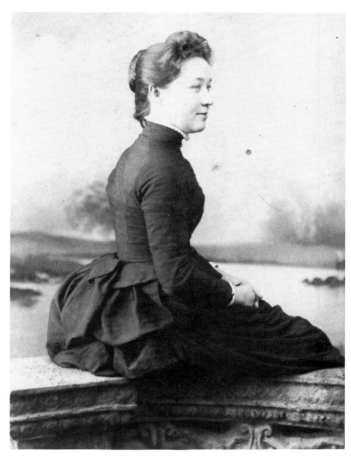

194

193.
Lady in extremely form-fitting basque bodice of woven-patterned satin with horizontally draped overskirt of a solid fabric.

194.
Seated woman in dress with bustle; high, round neckline.

195.
The man wears a finely checked suit with a four-button cutaway; bowler; cane. The woman is in a gown with a draped, pleated skirt with a bustle and the typical tight basque bodice; small hat; umbrella. A handkerchief is tucked under the bodice.

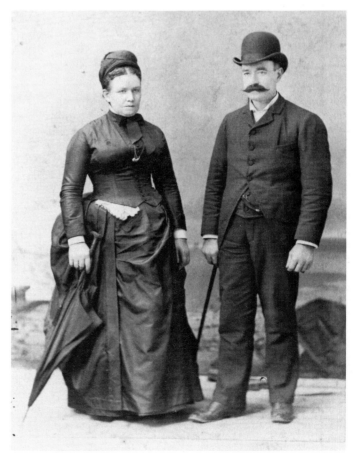

195

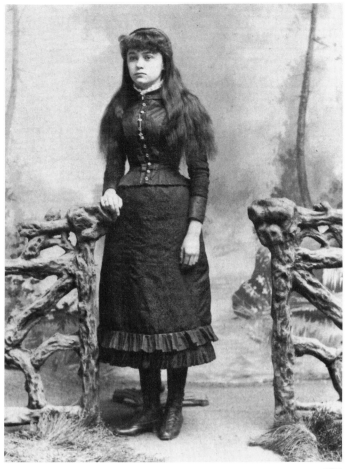

196

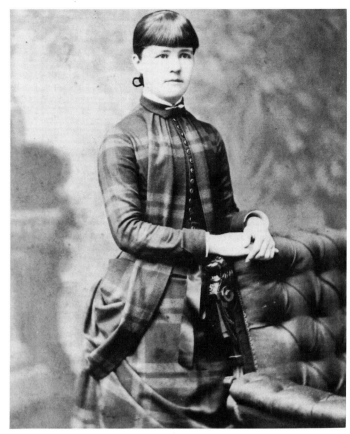

197

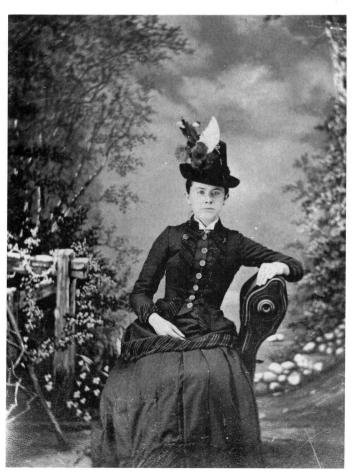

198

196.
Teenage girl in very tight, short basque; mid-calf skirt; long hair.

197.
Teenage girl in plaid wool dress with draped skirt and polonaise; spoon-shaped pin at high neck.

198.
High-crowned hat with birds' wings and plumes; gown with striped trim; pleated skirt.

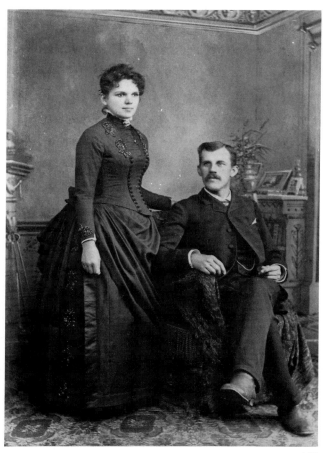

199

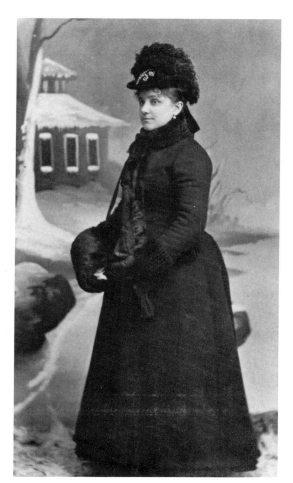

200

199.
The lady is in a tight basque with applied trim and decorative rows of buttons; draped and paneled skirt. The gentleman is in a three-piece, high-buttoned suit.

200.
A lady in winter coat cut to allow room for a bustle; muff; hat with plumes.

201.
Lady in rich self-patterned silk gown with a draped bustle over the pleated skirt; high neck with lace jabot; plumed hat.

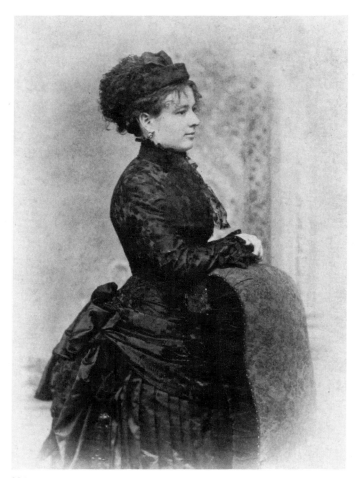

201

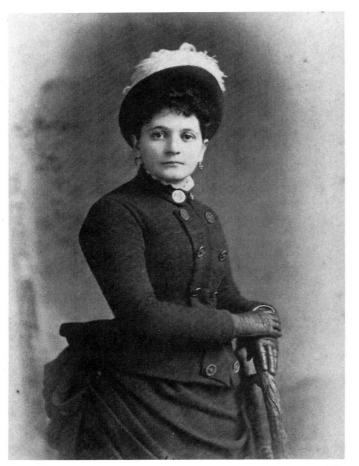

202

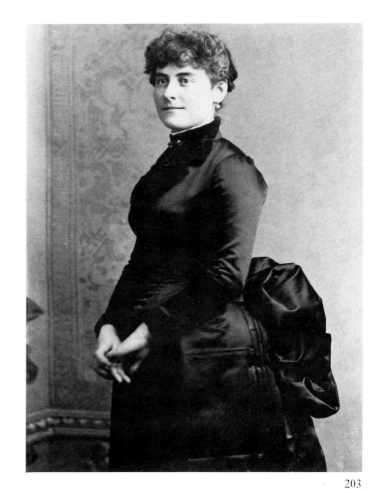

203

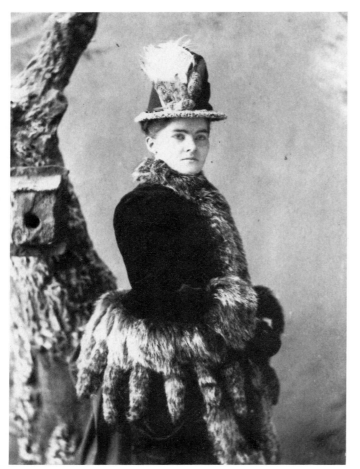

204

202.
Tailored wool double-breasted suit with extreme bustle; hat with white plumes.

203.
Heavy satin gown with high neck and huge pouf bustle.

204.
"Kate Lears, 1885." Flowerpot hat with birds' wings and plumes; mantle trimmed with fur and fur tails.

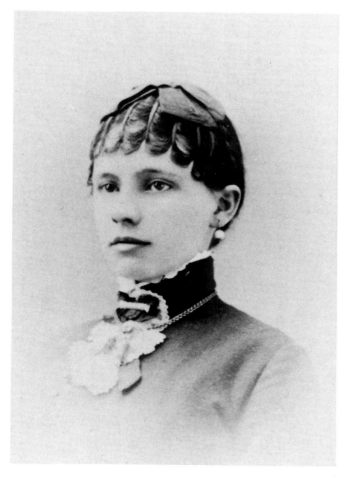

205

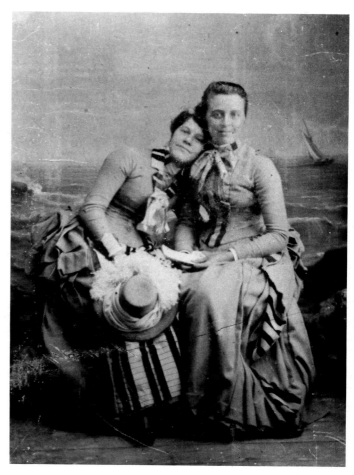

206

205.
Young woman with elaborate hairstyle featuring bangs looped through ribbons.

206.
Two women in similar (but not identical) dresses: striped, asymmetric trim; bustles; plumed hat.

207.
"Laura Knight," April 20, 1887. Another version of the bustle at its apex.

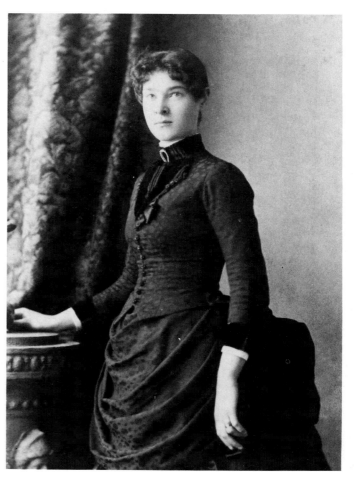

207

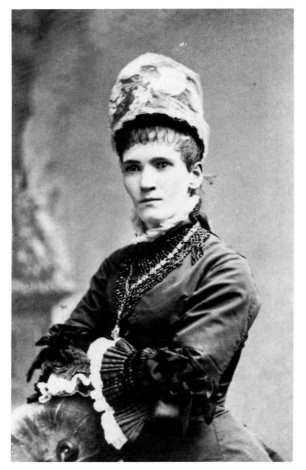

208

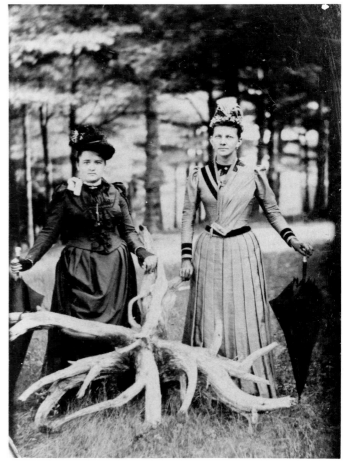

209

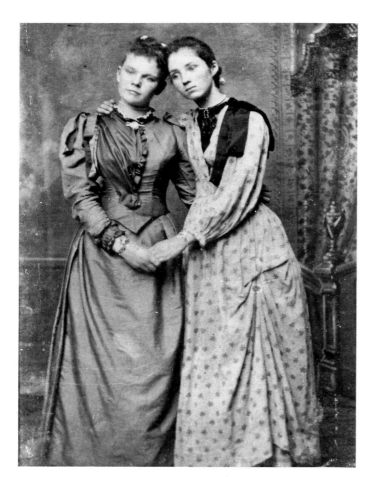

208.
Dress with jet trim on bodice; flaring, pleated, lace-trimmed cuffs; flowerpot hat with net and flowers; intricately looped bangs.

209.
Two ladies with umbrellas. The lady on the right wears a good example of the faddish asymmetric treatment of the bodice in the late eighties.

210.
In a sentimentally melancholy pose, both these young women wear gowns with contrasting material on one side of the bodice; the skirts are draped asymmetrically and there are no over-skirts.

210

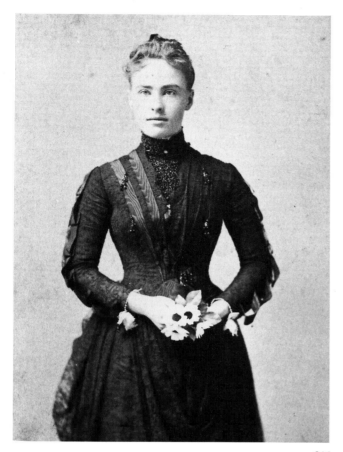

211

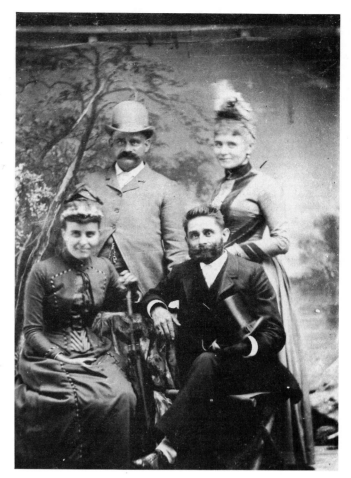

212

211.
Lace gown with teardrop jet trim; two parallel grosgrain ribbons trim one side of bodice; looped grosgrain trim on sleeves; high collar; dated 1888.

212.
"Nantasket [Massachusetts] Beach Aug 18, 1889, George & Kittie, Will & Rebecca just after a course dinner at the Atlantic House." The standing gentleman wears a three-button cutaway and bowler; the lady standing next to him shows off a fine figure in a dress with no perceptible bustle. The seated man holds a top hat; the seated lady, an umbrella.

213.
Lady with open lace-trimmed parasol; large hat with flowers; paisley-print gown with high neck, wide lapels, slightly puffed sleeves, and straight slim skirt with smocking detail.

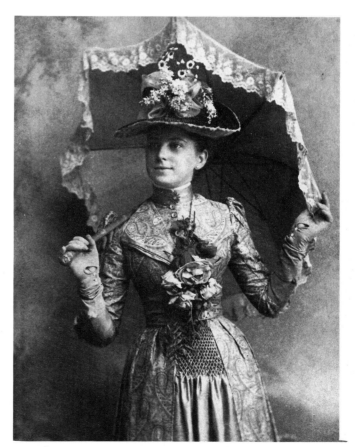

213

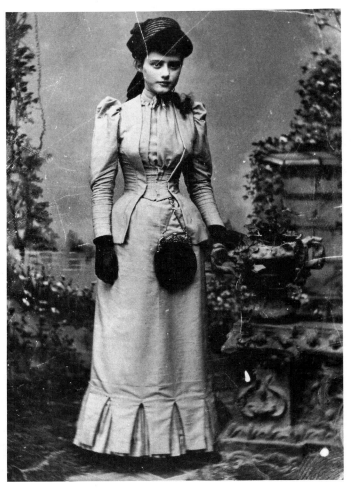

214

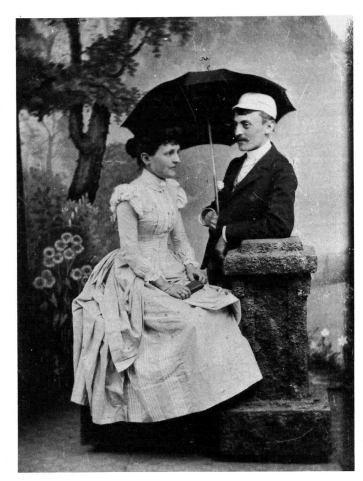

215

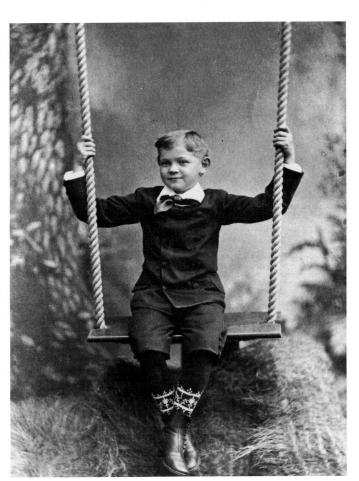

216

214.
Young woman with extremely tiny, tightly laced waist; slim skirt with godets at hem; slight rise at shoulders. The purse that hangs from a hook at the waist was known as a "chatelaine pocket."

215.
The woman wears a striped summer dress with the shoulder interest of the late eighties, although the draping, overskirt and rear fullness are more characteristic of the mid-eighties.

216.
"Walter Leigh, 1880." Double-breasted jacket, knee pants, patterned dark stockings, high-buttoned shoes.

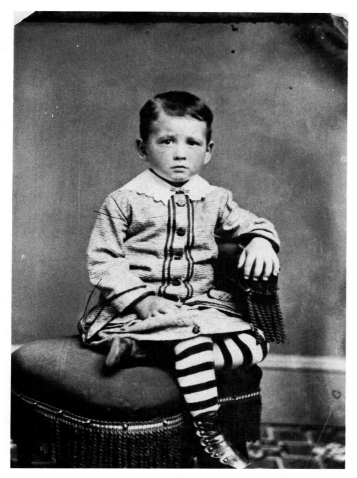

217

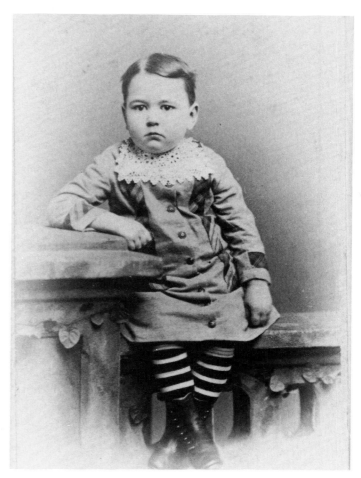

218

217.
Little boy in dress with lace collar; striped stockings.

218.
Another version of this popular style of dress for small boys features a wide, biblike lace collar; dated 1882.

219.
Girl in dress with tartan sash, scallops, pleats and lace jabot; grandfather in frock coat.

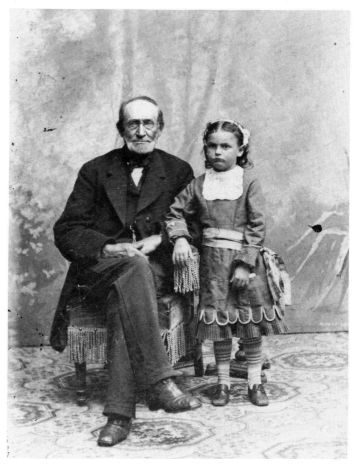

219

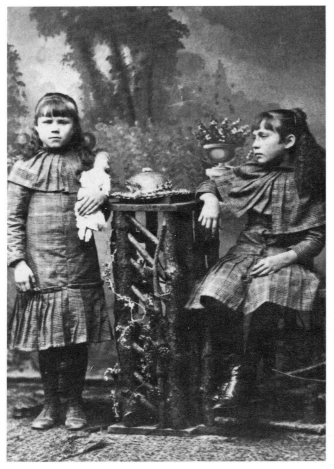

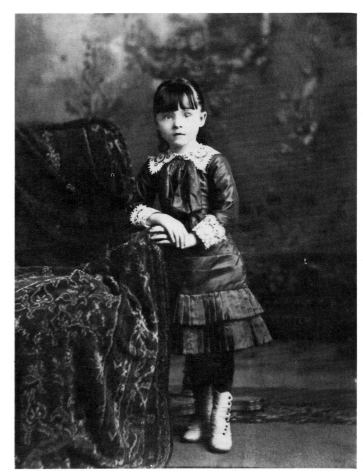

220

221

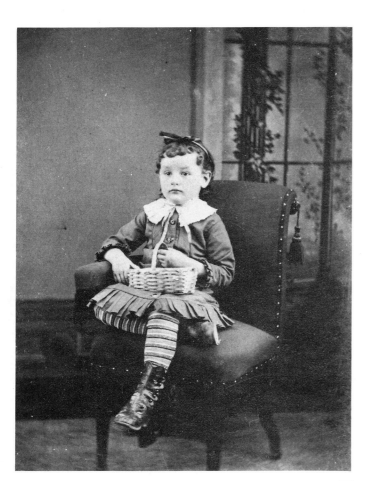

220.
Sisters in checked dresses with pleated cape-collars, no waists and deep, pleated hems; dated 1883.

221.
Girl in dress draped over the hips with two rows of pleated flounces at the hem; lace collar and cuffs; light-colored high buttoned shoes.

222.
Girl with basket. Her dress has pleats at the hem and cuffs; separate wide collar that ties in front; tricolored striped stockings.

222

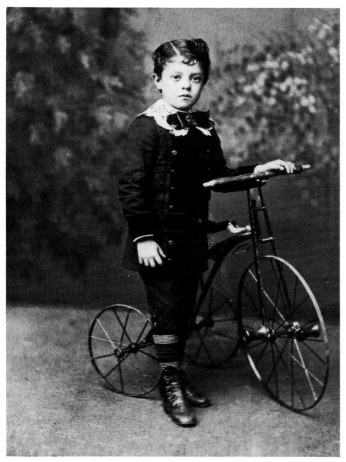

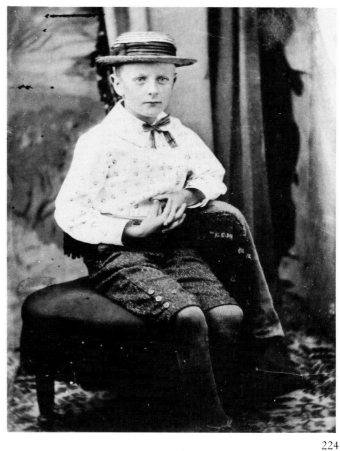

223

224

223.
"Guy T. Platt, Sacramento, Cal. Jan 1884." Low-waisted, belted jacket; knee pants; wide lace collar with large bow.

224.
"August 1885." Boy in print shirt, knee pants and straw hat.

225.
Even before *Little Lord Fauntleroy* became popular in 1886, party dress for boys generally included lace collar and cuffs and, sometimes, a sash as shown here.

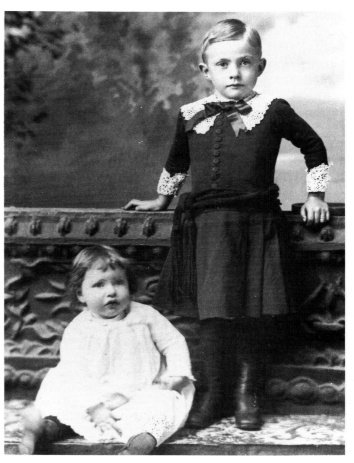

225

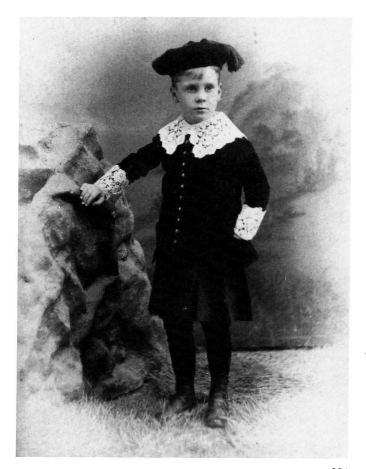

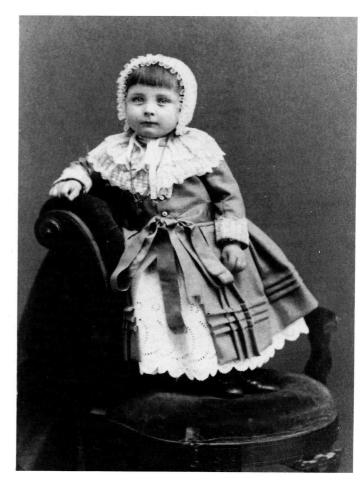

226

227

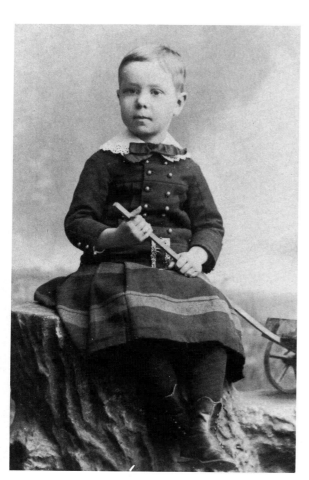

226.
Boy in Lord Fauntleroy velvet jacket and skirt. Very wide lace collar and cuffs; cavalier hat with tassel; dated 1886.

227.
Small girl in lightweight coat with satin-ribbon belt, opening over an eyelet dress; double lace bertha; lace cuffs; lace bonnet.

228.
Boy in a pleated, striped wool skirt and solid-color jacket; small lace collar with bow. Short hair was prevalent in this decade.

228

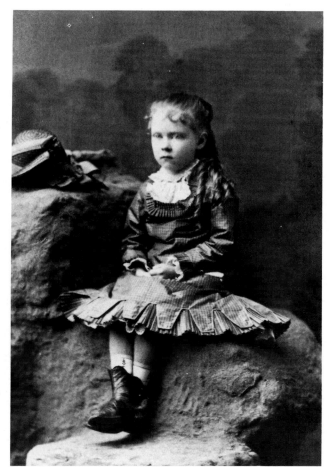

229

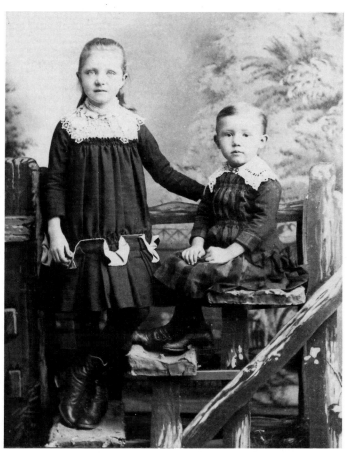

230

229.
A little girl with long curls wears a shiny, checked dress with pleated yoke and crenellated and pleated hem; socks with clocks.

230.
The girl wears a dress with fullness falling from the gathered yoke, contrast-trimmed, dropped waist. The boy wears a striped, gathered dress. Both have wide lace collars.

231.
Sisters in straw hats and dresses in identical print. Sash and dark mitts worn by girl on left; wide lace collar by girl on right.

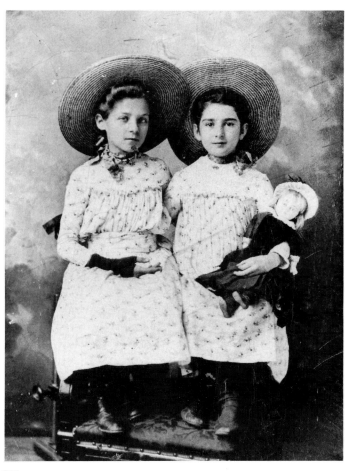

231

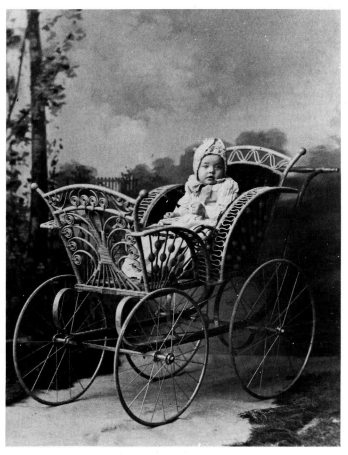

232

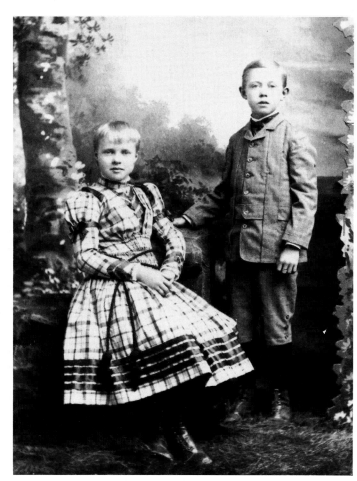

233

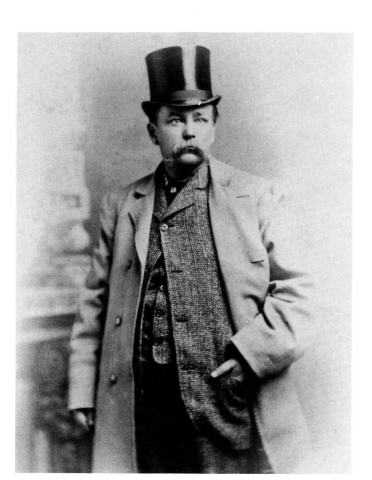

234

232.
A baby in a slightly pointed bonnet sits in a handsome wicker baby carriage.

233.
"Morton & Helen Wood, South Gardner Aug. 24–'89." She in plaid dress with bands of dark trim and slightly puffed upper sleeves; cord belt with tassels. He in Norfolk jacket and matching knee pants.

234.
Mustached gentleman in checked suit with top-buttoned coat; overcoat; top hat.

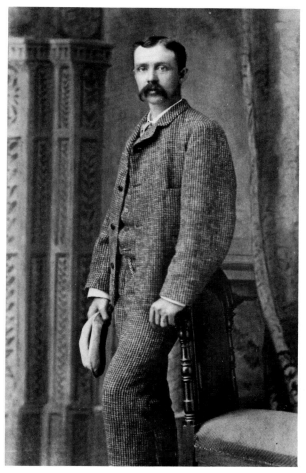

235

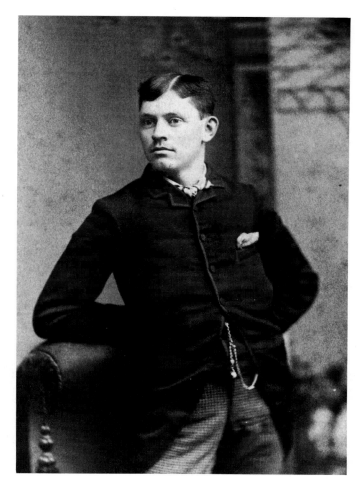

236

235.
Man in checked three-piece suit with very full sleeves; dated 1881.

236.
The stylish four-button cutaway worn with checked trousers.

237.
A windowpane-checked suit; stiff low collar and large four-in-hand tie.

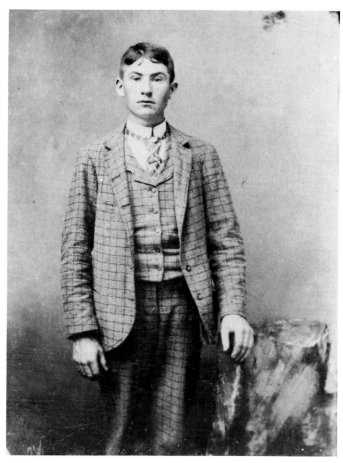

237

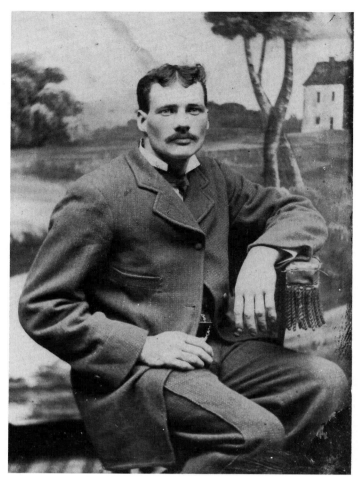

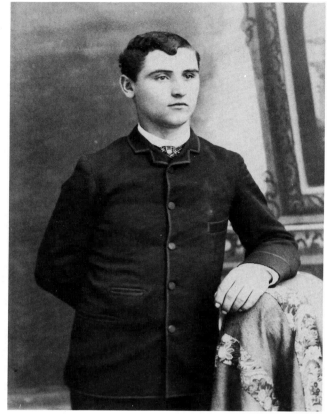

238

239

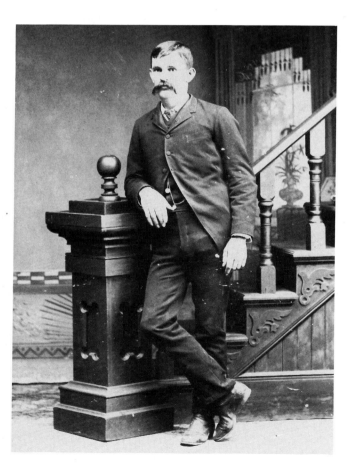

240

238.
Man with hair parted in center; heavy wool suit with high-buttoned coat; welted seam on trousers; wing collar.

239.
The tightly buttoned-up look in a narrow coat with very high neck and tiny lapels; three irregularly placed pockets.

240.
"Lela's father—Ruben Santee taken in Missouri about 1886." Three-button cutaway suit.

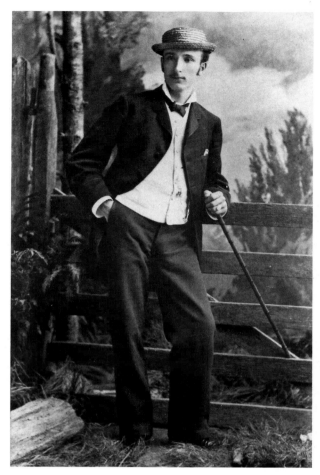

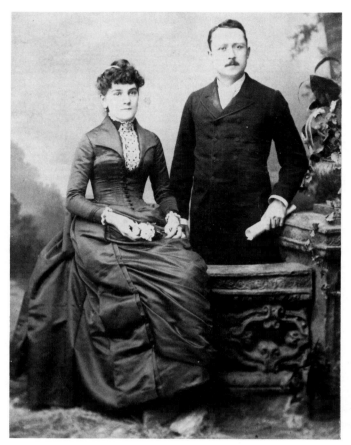

241

241.
Dapper man in light waistcoat, dark cutaway and trousers, wing collar, little bow tie, straw hat and cane.

242.
"Leou's father Samuel Walker"; "Dec. '87." A group of five men shows a variety of collars and ties, cutaway and high-buttoned coats, solid and checked trousers (those on the man far right showing mending on both legs). Four have mustaches; all have short hair.

243.
The gentleman wears a double-breasted frock coat with satin-faced lapels; white tie. The lady is in a silk dress with short basque bodice, draped skirt and back fullness.

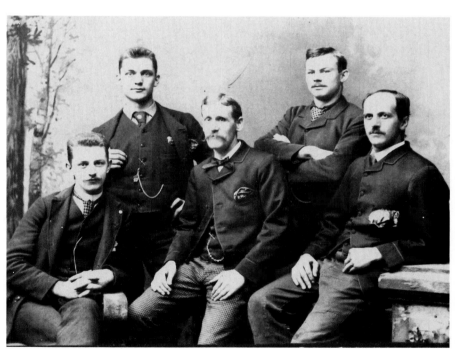

243

242

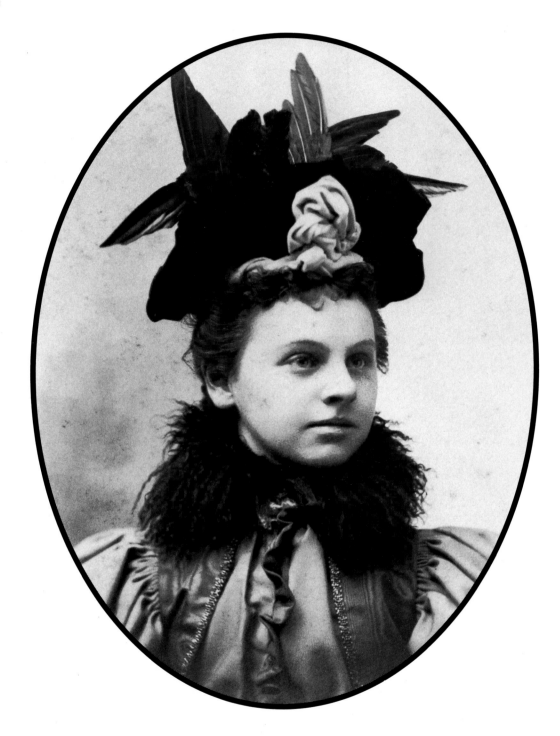

"Florence Dean." See Figure 247.

The 1890s

The flamboyant silhouette associated with the "Gay Nineties" took several years to evolve. The feeling at the start of the decade was much more restrained. A vestige of the bustle remained, and the skirts, quite narrow, continued to be somewhat gathered and draped. At first sleeves rose moderately at the shoulders, with the slight fullness of the upper arm tapering gradually to the wrist, but this trend quickly accelerated. By 1895 the delightfully exuberant nineties look was flourishing. Sleeves had grown so enormous and balloon-like that they sometimes had to be supported by linings of stiffened muslin or taffeta. (As in the days of the hoopskirt, the ultrafashionable lady once again might have a problem getting through a doorway.) From the tiny corseted waist a plain gored skirt flared out gracefully and, thanks to its taffeta lining, rustled enticingly when in motion. The only escape from the high, boned collar was in evening dress, in which low necklines and trains were seen. Fabrics were opulent and colors bright.

Hair was worn up, usually off the forehead. The bonnet had almost disappeared, and its remaining adherents were apt to be well along in years. Sizable hats were generously heaped with stiff bows, flowers, lace, ribbons, feathers and birds, in various imaginative arrangements. One impressive model, worn squarely on top of the head, bristled with several tall individual plumes in a most formidable manner. Understatement was not in vogue.

This was also the era of the separate skirt and shirtwaist, now available ready-made and beloved by the increasing numbers of young women entering the workforce in sales and office positions. The many different outfits that could be created with just a few blouses and skirts made a limited wardrobe appear much more extensive. This tailored look, made even more popular in the late nineties by the Gibson Girl, was rescued from complete practicality by its firm adherence to whatever sleeve size was currently stylish. At the same time, a very masculine four-in-hand or bow tie might be worn at the neck, and belts were ubiquitous. In summer such a costume was often topped by a straw boater that was indistinguishable from the male version.

Also borrowed from the gentlemen was the very popular tailored suit, with a version appropriate for almost any activity a woman might be interested in. An advertisement in *Munsey's Magazine* of June 1896 offered "Outing, Golf, Cycle, Tennis, Travelling, Walking and Wash Suits" (p. 385). Another advertisement in the same issue, reflecting the current craze for bicycling, promoted a five-piece outfit of blazer, knickerbockers, skirt, cap and leggings, and featuring, of course, the contemporary huge sleeve.

As the nineties waned, the sleeve did, too. Epaulets and very exaggerated, wide collars now provided the interest. Skirts were narrower and very slim over the hips, but still swirled elegantly at the hemline. The bodice was frequently emphasized with lace. Some gloriously large and overdecorated hats were to be seen.

Men's sack, or lounge, suits, with moderately broad collar and lapels, had lost the tightly buttoned-up look of the eighties and look relatively modern. They were generally worn with wing or turned-down collars, and the four-in-hand tie had established its supremacy, although pre-tied ascot and modest bow ties were still in the picture. Trousers might have creases and cuffs. The derby (or bowler), the homburg, the straw boater and the top hat all had a place in the well-dressed man's wardrobe. Belted Norfolk jackets and knickerbockers were popular for sports and bicycling—the latter the rage for both sexes in the nineties.

In children's clothes, the extreme length of younger boys' and girls' dresses is most striking. Girls' dresses and coats often had a cape effect at the shoulders, and the size of the sleeve followed the current fashion. Hair was frequently shoulder-length and curly; bangs were not as universal as they had been in the eighties. The youngest boys might also have full sleeves like their mothers', while slightly older boys often wore pleated skirts with middy blouses or jackets. The *Ladies' Home Journal* of August 1893 said, "Put a well-grown boy of four years in knee trousers, with round, and Eton jackets and blouses" (p. 29), but not all boys were lucky enough to be out of skirts so young. A wide, soft scarf, tied in a big bow, dressed up the knee pants and jacket outfits, although for special occasions the Little Lord Fauntleroy lace-and-velvet look had lost none of its appeal. The sailor suit also remained a favorite. Striped stockings had vanished, replaced by solid-color dark ones (sometimes white for younger children) and high-buttoned shoes or boots were worn almost exclusively.

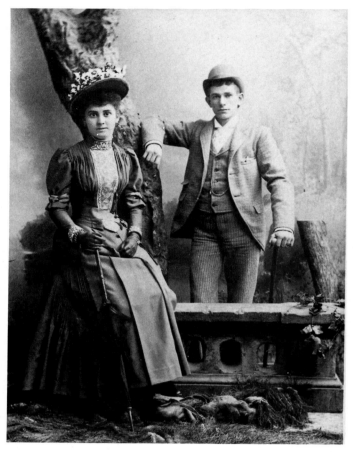

244

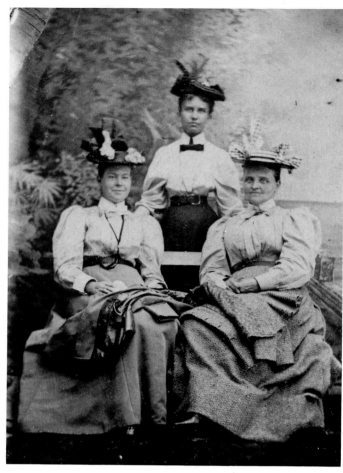

245

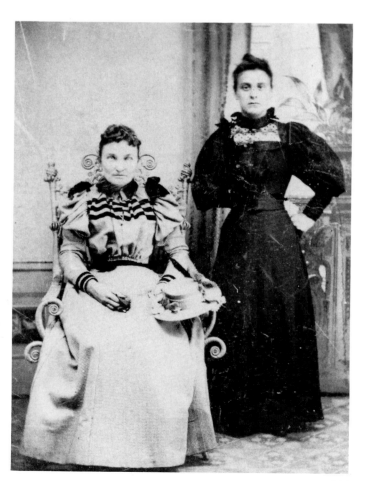

246

244.
The lady's shirred bodice opens over a decorative plastron; the skirt is box-pleated; slightly puffed upper sleeves. He wears a checked jacket with matching vest, striped trousers and a bowler.

245.
These three ladies wear wool tailormades, shirtwaists with full sleeves, stiff, high collars, mannish bow ties, belts and shallow-crowned hats with ribbons and feathers.

246.
The lady on the left wears a finely checked dress with dark trim on the bodice, plain skirt, moderate sleeves. (Wicker "curls" of the chair frame her head.) Her companion has larger sleeves.

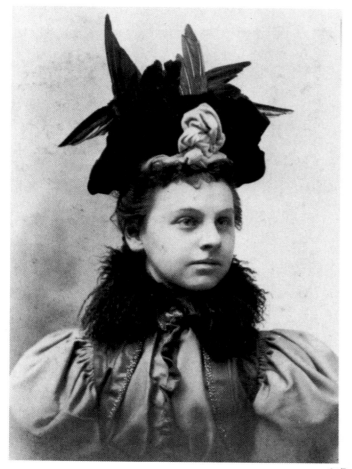

247

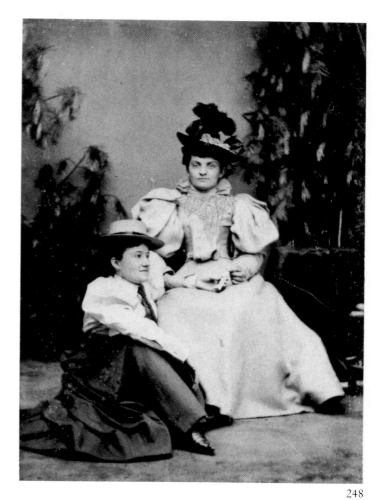

248

247.
"Florence Dean." Velvet hat with birds' wings; ostrich collar.

248.
Seated on the floor, a woman in shirtwaist and skirt, four-in-hand tie and boater, daringly offers a pack of cigarettes to a friend whose outfit includes a lace-encrusted bodice, neck ruff, huge sleeves, plain gored skirt and large plumed hat.

249.
All four ladies wear shirtwaists with plain belted skirts; their hats range from boaters with birds' wings to larger creations with flowers and ostrich plumes.

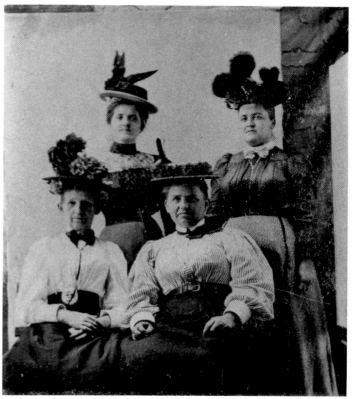

249

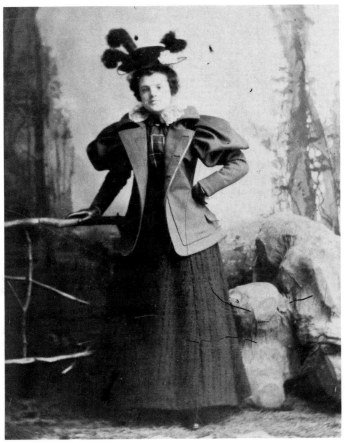

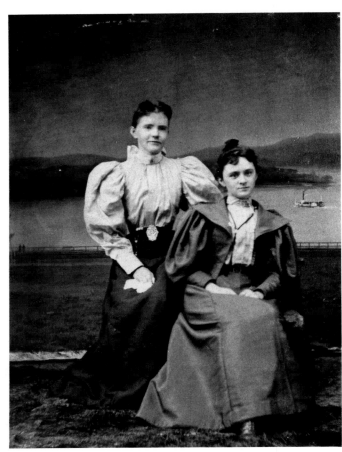

250

251

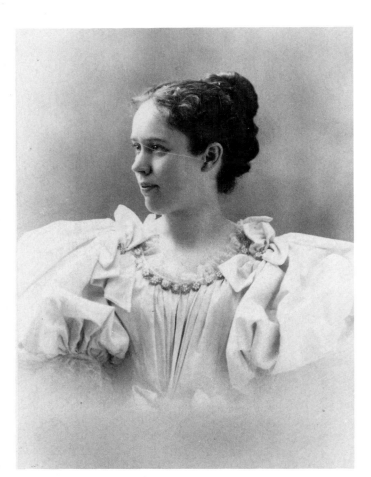

250.
A lighthearted effect is created by the huge-sleeved, wide-lapelled, fitted jacket, ankle-length skirt and a hat with jaunty plumes.

251.
The woman on the left wears a full-sleeved blouse with a big bow at back of neck. The woman on the right wears a suit jacket with wide lapels and leg-o'-mutton sleeves. Both have plain skirts.

252.
Young woman in dinner gown with round neck trimmed with clusters of seed pearls; huge melon sleeves topped with bows.

252

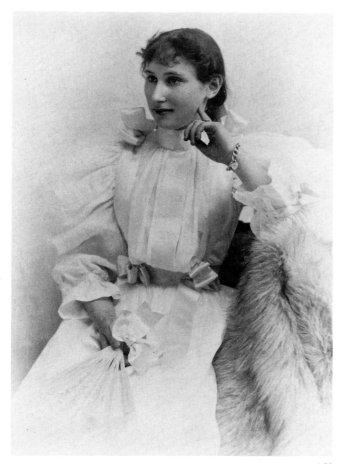

253

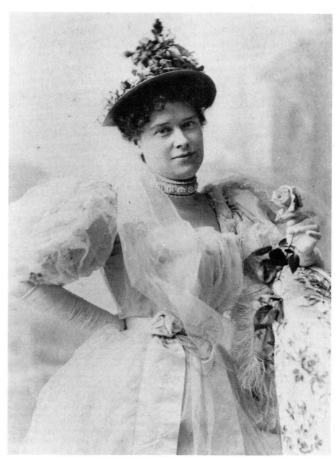

254

253.
"Mae Irvin, Englishtown NJ." A delicate gown with large sleeves, satin ribbon belt, bows, high boned collar; fan.

254.
Lady holding a rose. Dress with gauzy sleeves, square neckline; seed-pearl choker, elbow-length gloves, hat.

255.
Evelyn Betts, the author's grandmother-in-law, strikes a romantic pose in a mid-nineties dinner dress with enormous sleeves and a lace-, ribbon- and flower-trimmed neckline.

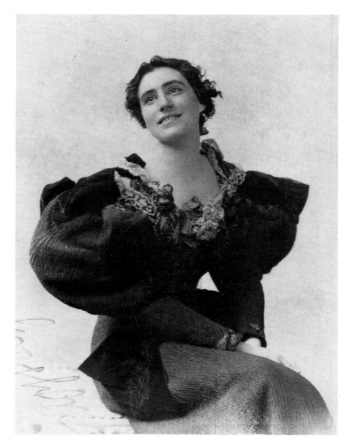

255

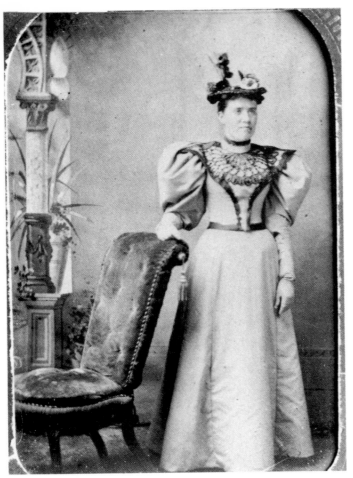

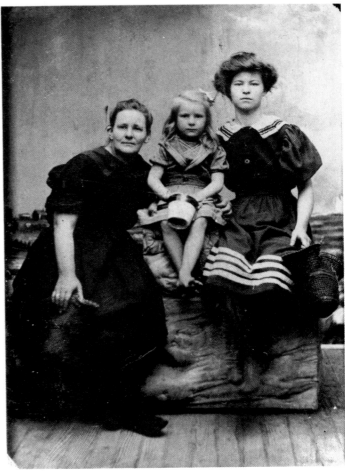

256

258

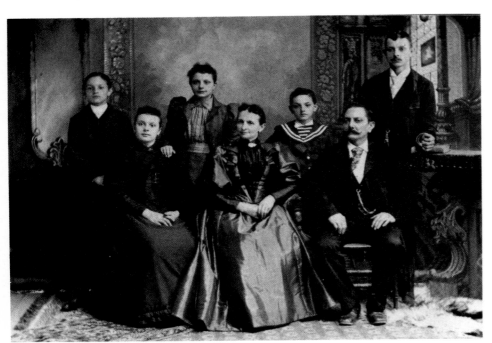

257

256.
Visiting dress in heavy, pale silk with decorated bodice, leg-o'-mutton sleeves and plain gored skirt. The hat, with flowers and aigrettes, sits squarely on the head.

257.
A family portrait, the matriarch in glistening taffeta with large sleeves and cascading lapels, the father in a three-piece suit with four-in-hand tie, the youngest boy in a sailor suit.

258.
A trio of bathers. The women are in stockings and hold high-crowned, floppy straw hats.

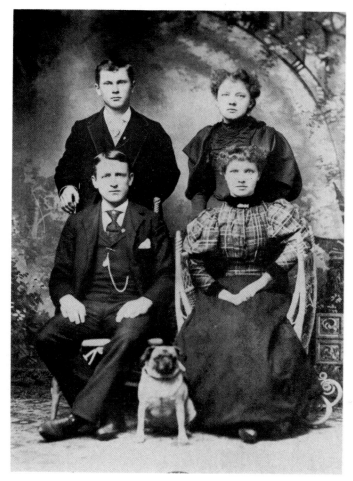

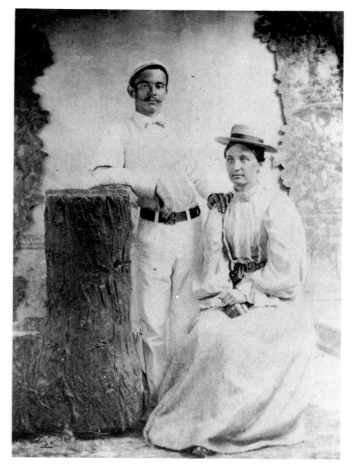

259

261

259.
The tight, high-buttoned look of men's clothes of the eighties has virtually vanished and an easier, quite modern feeling has replaced it. The ladies have typical mid-nineties sleeves.

260.
A family group. The boy on the right wears a heavy pleated skirt and matching top with middy collar; the boy on the left is in the same heavy material in a dress with leg-o'-mutton sleeves like his mother's. The father is in a three-piece suit, four-in-hand tie.

261.
A couple in sports clothes. The young woman is in a full-sleeved, lightweight shirtwaist, plain skirt and straw boater. The man is in his shirt sleeves, with bow tie and cap. Noteworthy are his trousers with loops for the belt—new in this decade.

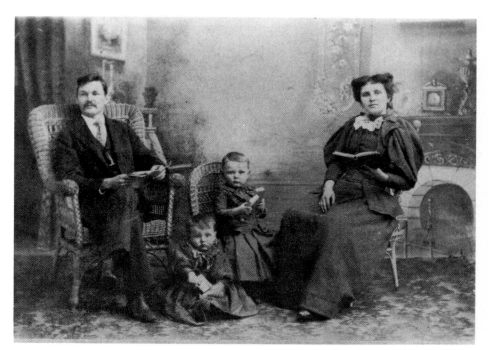

260

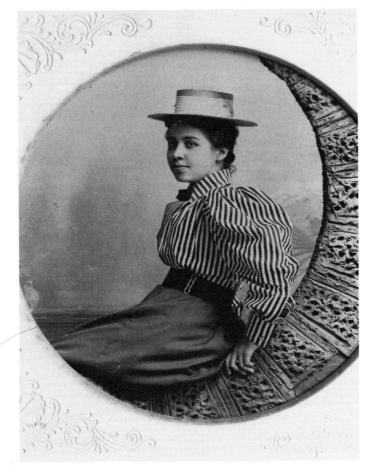

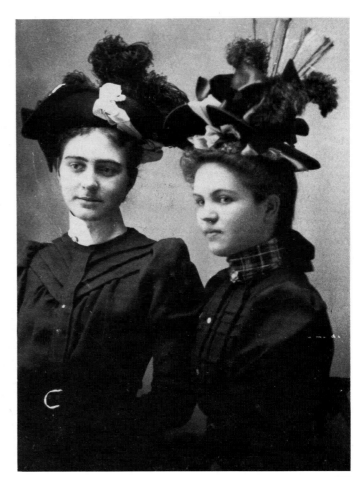

262

263

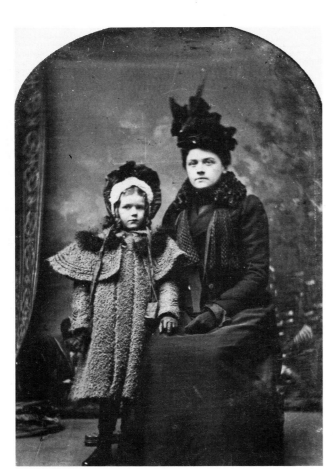

262.
"G.A. Goodhue, B.H.S. '97." Young woman in striped shirtwaist and straw boater.

263.
"Carrie MacIsaac Kittie Doome Feb. 1899 Prov. R.I." Unforgettable hats—plumes, aigrettes and ribbon. Their sleeves have only the slightest rise at the shoulders.

264.
"Gertie and Anna Wish you a happy New Year." Girl in textured-wool fur-trimmed coat with shoulder cape; high-crowned bonnet. Lady in fur-trimmed coat; high-crowned toque with a aigrette and ribbons.

264

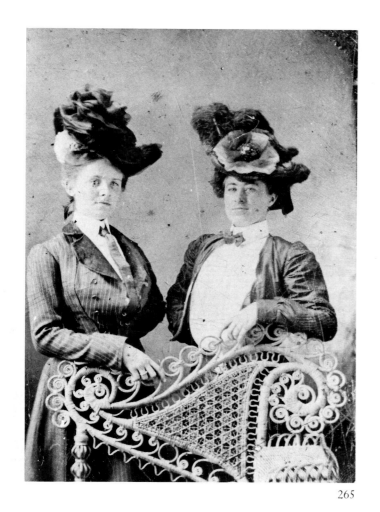

265

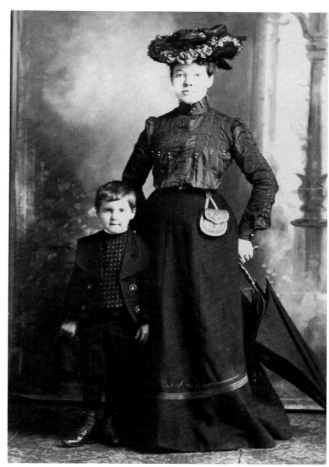

266

265.
Two women in late nineties tailored suits, Gibson Girl shirtwaists with stiff collars, ties and huge, incongruous, flower-laden hats.

266.
Woman in high-necked shirtwaist with pleated tabs and pearl decoration; flared wool skirt with slight train; chatelaine purse at waist; large, flowered hat; umbrella. The little boy is in knee pants, a jacket with very wide lapels and knitted sweater.

267.
Little girl in long dress with smocked yoke, full-sleeved blouse. Little boy in suit with some sleeve fullness, striped middy collar, knees with buckle-and-button trim; tam-o'-shanter; identical hair-styles for both children.

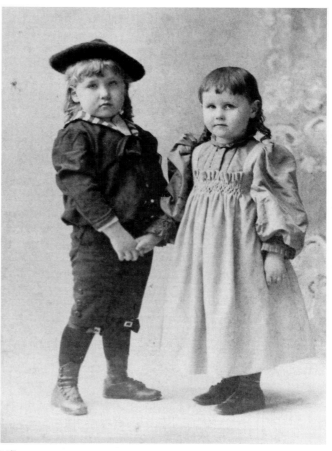

267

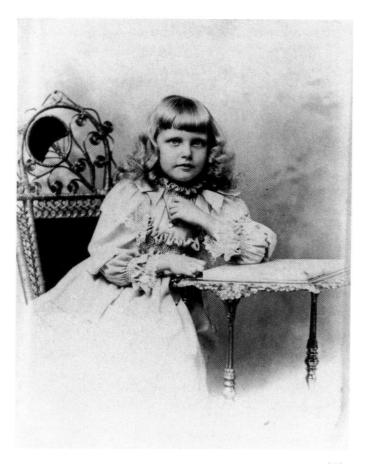

268

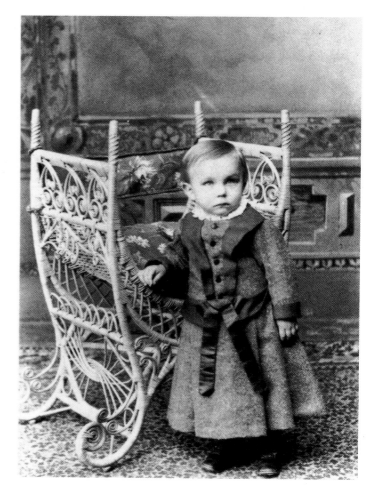

269

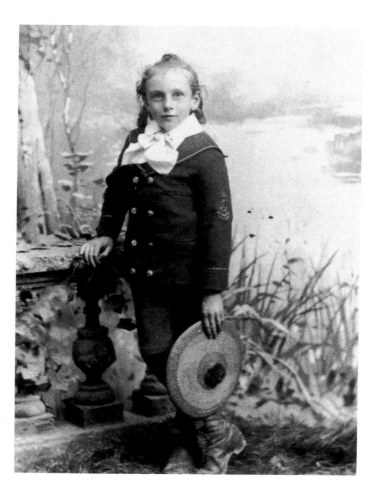

270

268.
Dress with the soft ruffles, lace and smocking of the early nineties.

269.
Little boy in long wool dress with satin trim and small lace collar.

270.
Sailor suit with knee pants, worn with a big bow at the neck, long curls; dated 1892.

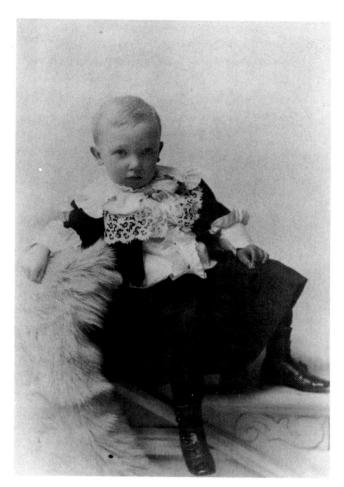

271

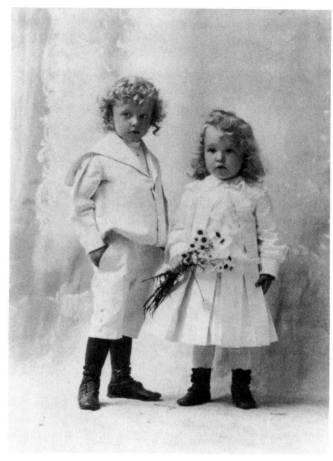

272

271.
The Little Lord Fauntleroy influence lingered on through the nineties. Despite skirt, lace and ruffles, this boy manages to retain a very masculine appearance.

272.
"Bulkely Smith——4 years July 3 Willard Smith 2 years 8 mos June 1895." The elder boy is in a sailor suit with middy blouse and knee pants; the younger wears a box-pleated skirt and frilly blouse.

273.
Little boy in Lord Fauntleroy outfit with knee pants and an exceptionally wide, lacy collar.

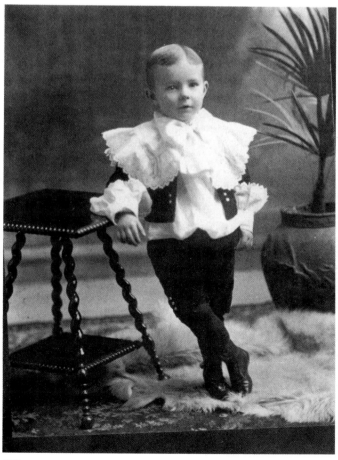

273

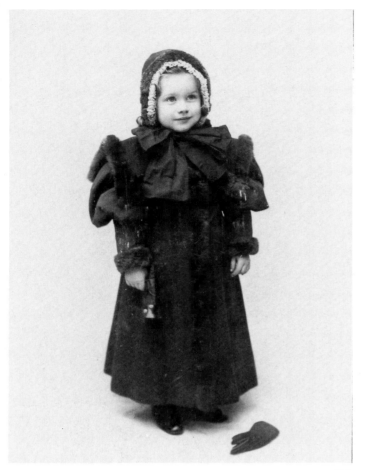

274

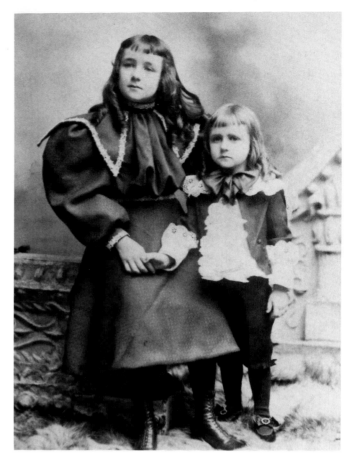

275

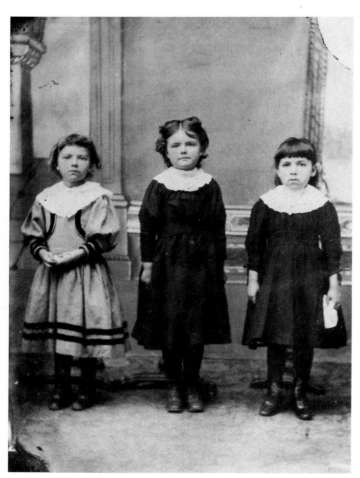

276

274.
"Violetta I. Taff Four years old." Leg-o'-mutton-sleeved, fur-trimmed, ankle-length coat and fur-trimmed bonnet with very wide ribbons.

275.
Girl in dress with voluminous sleeves, exaggerated cape collar and plain skirt. Her little brother wears Lord Fauntleroy suit of knee pants, frilly blouse and low shoes with bows and buckles. Both have bangs and long corkscrew curls.

276.
Three girls in varying degrees of sleeve fullness. All wear very wide, detachable, washable collars, black stockings, high-buttoned shoes.

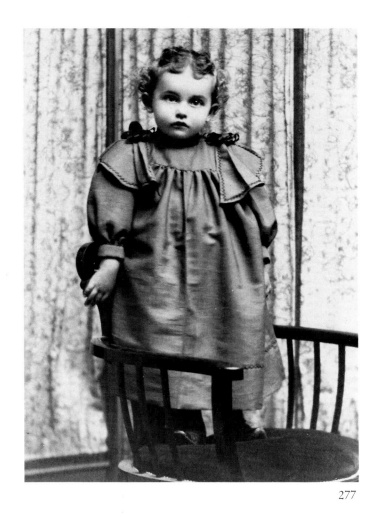

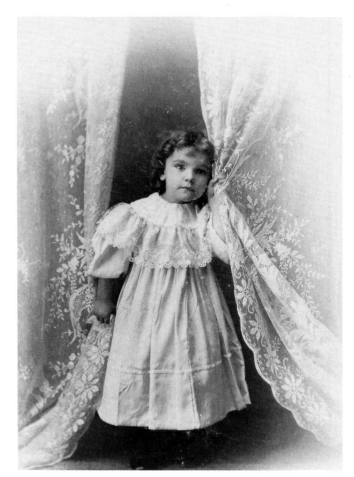

277

278

277.
Little girl with moderate sleeves, bows and cape effect at shoulders; ankle-length dress.

278.
Little girl in long lightweight dress with wide lace bertha giving a cape effect. Embroidered net curtains.

279.
A missing button and somewhat droopy leg-o'-mutton sleeves give a hand-me-down air to this little girl's oversized wool coat.

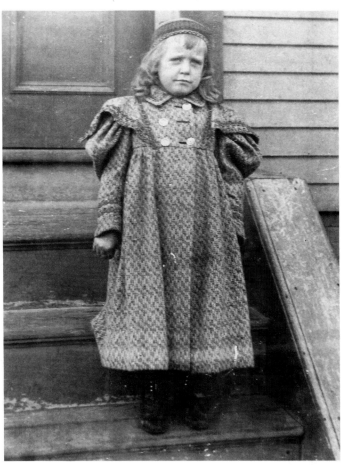

279

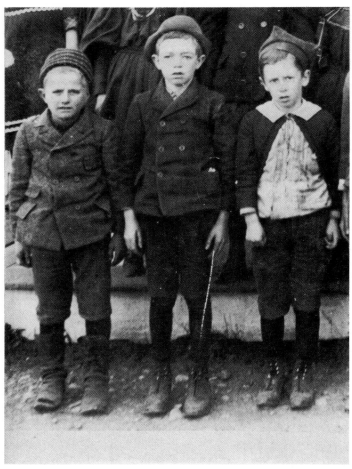

280

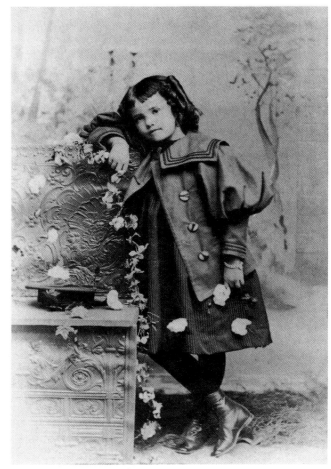

281

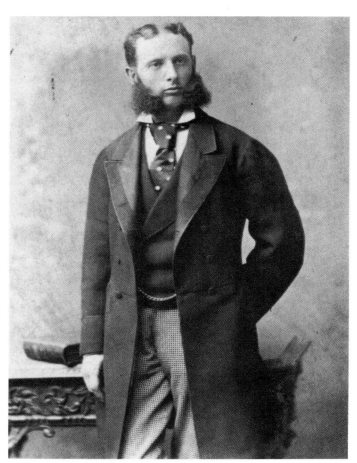

282

280.
Detail, class picture, 1896. The ragtag appearance of these three boys, in their knee pants, outgrown jackets and well-worn boots, was undoubtedly a much more common sight in this decade than the velvet-and-lace look.

281.
Girl in striped dress and jacket with square collar and leg-o'-mutton sleeves; three parallel rows of braid trim on collar and cuffs.

282.
Frock coat with silk-faced lapels, worn with matching vest and finely checked trousers. The big polka-dot tie, worn here with a wing collar, was particularly popular in the nineties. Mutton-chop whiskers.

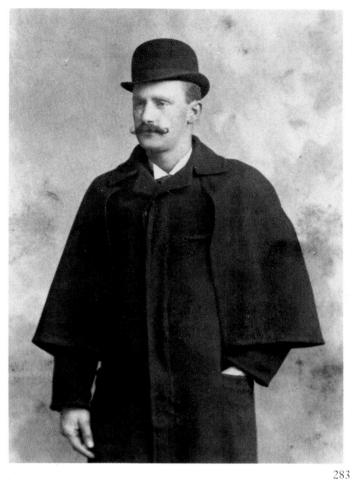

283

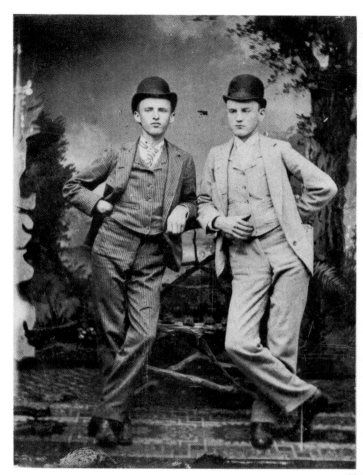

284

283.
"Taken before 1896 Frank MacDavitt, Lynn, Mass." Inverness coat.

284.
These three-piece lounge suits include vests with four pockets; bowlers.

285.
The cummerbund and trousers with cuffs seen on the left were current novelties, as were the creased trousers on the right.

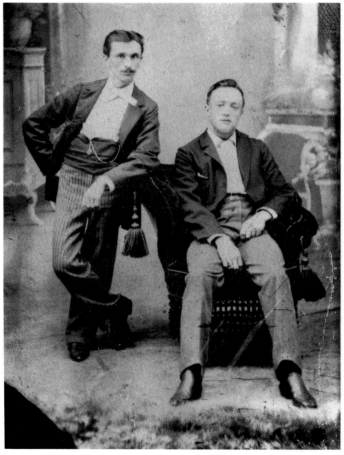

285

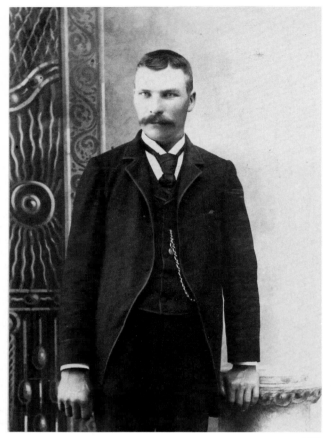

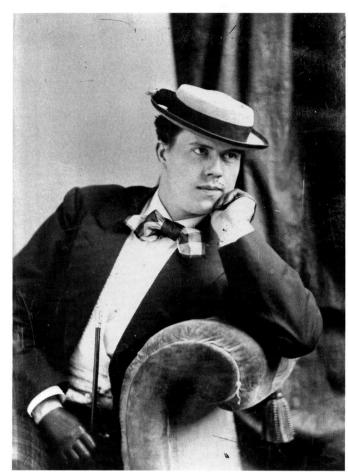

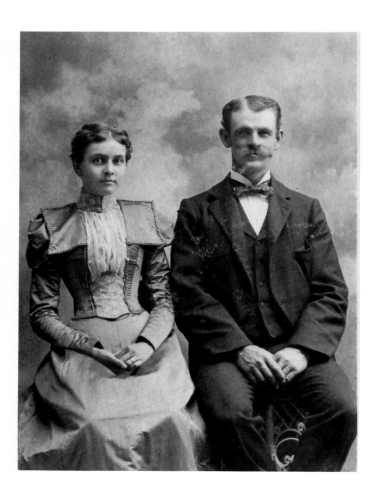

286.
Man in morning coat, wing collar, big tie. An 1894 *Harper's Weekly* illustration of the New York Stock Exchange shows many of the brokers in similar attire.

287.
Dapper gentleman wearing straw porkpie hat at a rakish angle, big checked bow tie, white vest, dark jacket and gloves.

288.
The young woman's very high, boned collar, wide lapels and diminished sleeves are characteristic of the late nineties. Her husband shows that, despite differences in cut, the general appearance of men's suits has not changed drastically over the ensuing years.

Notes on the Images

The following notes list the technique or format of the images reproduced, as well as certain information written or printed on the photograph or its mount. The following abbreviations are used: D (daguerreotype; 1839–ca. 1860, the examples in this work dating from the 1840s and 1850s); A (ambrotype; 1854–ca. 1865); T (tintype; 1856 on); V (carte de visite; 1860–1880s); C (cabinet card; 1866 on, the examples in this book dating from 1870 on). The numbers are those of the figures.

The 1840s

All images are daguerreotypes. **9:** "Higgins." **20:** "Van Loan Gallery, 158 Chestnut St., Philada." **24:** "Atkins."

The 1850s

25–29: D. **30:** D; "Carleton, Artist, Portland, Me." **31–34:** D. **35:** T. **36:** A. **37:** T. **38–40:** A. **41:** A; "Hazelton's Photograph Rooms, 385 Washington Street, Boston. Few doors South of Boston Theatre. Ambrotypes 12½ cents. Likenesses set in lockets, pins, and fancy cases. Copying neatly & carefully executed. Sick and Deceased Persons taken at their residences." **42:** T. **43:** A; "Price List of the National Daguerrian Gallery, 103 Court Street, Branch of the Mammoth Daguerrian Rooms, 228 Washington, corner Summer Street, J. D. Heywood, Proprietor," ambrotypes and daguerreotypes being advertised at "$.25, .50, $1.00, 1.25, 1.50, 2.00, 3.00, 5.00, 10.00." **44, 45:** T. **46, 47:** D. **48:** A. **49:** D. **50:** T; "Melainotype plate for Neff's pat 19 Feb 56." **51:** D. **52:** T. **53:** D. **54:** A. **55–57:** T.

The 1860s

58: V; "K. W. Beniczky, Photographer, No 2 New Chambers St Cor. Chatham St., NY." **59:** V; "Jaquith, 167 Broadway." **60:** V. **61:** V; "B. Whiting, 16 Main St., Plymouth, Mass." **62:** V; "W. Snell, 188 Essex St., Salem." **63:** V; "J. N. Hardenbrook, photographer, 74 Prince William St. St. John, N. B." **64:** V; "K. W. Beniczky, Photographer, No 2 New Chambers St Cor. Chatham St., NY." **65:** V. **66:** V; "Gorham & Co., 12 Steeple St., Providence, R. I." **67:** T. **68:** V. **69:** V; "Died Nov 11/63 Wednesday Evening"; "Dunshee, Artist, 175 Westminster St., Providence, R. I." **70, 71:** T. **72:** V; red five-cent revenue stamp of 1864–66. **73:** V; "Warren—Lowell & Cambridgeport." **74:** V; "B. Carr & Co., Concord, N. H." **75:** T. **76:** V; blue two-cent revenue stamp of 1864–66. **77:** T. **78:** V. **79:** V; "M. Smith, No. 134½ Union St., New Bedford." **80:** V; "W. H. Sherman, Photographer, 385 Main St., Milwaukee." **81:** T. **82–87:** T. **88:** V; "Photographed by A. A. Watson, 87 King St., St. John, N. B.

Copies of this can be had at any time." **89:** V. **90:** V; "Harley, Metcalf & Winter, Photographers, Harvard Square, Cambridge." **91:** V; "Howard, Parisian Photographer, ½ Purchase St., New Bedford, Mass. Negatives Preserved." **92:** T; "Bolles & Frisbie, Photographers, Gallery No. 3, Bank Street, New London, Conn." **93:** V; "Silsbee, Case & Co. Photograph Artists, 299½ Washington St., Boston." **94, 95:** T. **96:** A. **97:** V; "C. Seaver, Jr. Photographer, 27 Tremont Row, Boston." **98:** T. **99:** V; "to Mary—from Cousin Christina"; "Chisholm, Photographer, St. Johns, N. F." **100:** V. **101:** V; "Hart's Arcade Photographic Gallery, Watertown, N. Y." **102:** T. **103:** V; "A. C. Nichols, Photographer, Leavenworth, Kansas." **104:** V. **105:** V; "W. H. Jennings, Cor Main & Shetucket Sts., Norwich, Ct. Additional Copies of this picture may be obtained by sending the name." **106:** T; "Bolles & Frisbie's New Style of Pictures, Taken and Delivered in 15 Minutes, Can only be obtained at our Gallery, No. 4 Bank Street, New London, Ct. The Largest Assortment of Photograph Frames In the City. For sale at Our Gallery." **107:** V; "Lydston, Artist and Photographer, Cor. Wis. & Main Sts., Milwaukee"; green three-cent revenue stamp of 1865. **108:** V; "S.H. Waite, Photographer, 275 Main St., Hartford, Conn." **109:** V; A.D. Terhune, Photographer, Hackensack, N.J. Duplicates of this Picture can be had at any time." **110, 111:** V; "J.H. Nolan, Photographer, Waterville, N. Y. Pictures will be made from this negative at any time when they are ordered during the year 1867." **112:** V. **113:** V; "H. K. Averill, Jr., Plattsburgh, N.Y." **114:** V; "C.D. Fredericks & Co., 587 Broadway, New York, —— de la Habana, Habana, 31 Passage du Havre, Paris." **115, 116:** T. **117:** T; "A.E. Alden's New Style Carte de Visite, By Machinery, 16 Tintypes for 25¢, Two Positions given and a Present to each customer. At the Arcade Gallery, Nos. 60 & 62 in Arcade, Providence, R. I."; blue two-cent revenue stamp of 1864–66. **118:** V; "D.T. Burrell, Photographer, Bridgewater, Mass."; green three-cent revenue stamp of 1864–66. **119:** V; "C.L. Pond's Photograph Gallery, No. 204 Main Street, Buffalo." **120:** V. **121:** T. **122:** T. **123:** V.

The 1870s

124–135: T. **136:** V; "Audaciter, Ewing Photo, [by appointment?] to H.R.H. Prince Arthur." **137:** V; "Sarony & Co., Photographers, 680 Broadway, N.Y. Napoleon Sarony, Alfred S. Campbell." **138–140:** T. **141:** C; "North & Oswald, Portrait & Landscape Photographers, New Studios, 32 & 33 Finlay's Chamber of Commerce, Toledo, O." **142:** C; "D. B. Vickery, Haverhill, Mass." **143:** V; "Slee Bros, Photographers, Po'keepsie, N.Y." **144:** T. **145:** C; "Isaac White, No. 15 Pratt St., Hartford, Conn." **146:** C; "D. K. Prescott, Tremont Row, Boston, Loomis Gallery"; "To my sincere friend Harry B —— From his —— John —— H——." **147:** C; "W. G. Chamberlain, Cor. Larimer & Fifteenth Streets, Denver. Visitors are invited to examine our Stereoscopic Views of Colorado Scenery, of which we have a very extensive and interesting collection." **148:** T. **149:**

C; "Steckel, 220 S. Spring St., Los Angeles, Cal." **150:** C; "From the Studio of Chas H. Lindsey, Photographer, Murgatroyd's Block, Nashua, N.H." **151-154:** T. **155:** C; "Caton, Post Office Block, Manchester, N. H." **156:** "Yosemite Art Gallery, I. W. Taber & T. H. Boyd, 26 Montg'y St., San Francisco, Cal'a. I. W. Taber & Co." **157, 158:** T. **159:** V; "James Inglis, Photographer, Montreal." **160, 161:** T. **162:** V; " 'Berlin Photograph' by A. J. Jackson, Photographer, Rockland, Me." **163:** V; "The Saratoga Photograph Co., Ground Floor Gallery, 197 Broadway, Saratoga Springs Myers, Manager." **164:** T. **165:** V; "J. H. Lamson Photographer, 152 Middle Street, Portland, Maine." **166, 167:** T. **168:** V; "Edouart's Enameled Cards, Kearny, corner California [Streets, San Francisco]." **169-172:** T. **173:** V; "——. F. Keniston 355½ Main St., Fitchburg, Mass." **174:** V; "Blessing & Bro. Photographers, 174 Tremont Street, Galveston, Texas. Send name and get additional prints, at $3 per dozen." **175-178:** T. **179:** V; "G. W. Wood & Co, Photographers, Cor. Washington & Michigan Aves., Lansing, Mich." **180-183:** T.

The 1880s

184: C; "W. H. Abbott, Photographer, Little Falls, NY   Duplicates kept for further orders." **185, 186:** T. **187:** C. **188:** V; "P. L. Brault, Artiste, Photographe, 131 Rue Richelieu, St. Jean, P. Q." **189:** T. **190:** C; "Chickering, 21 West St., Boston." **191:** C; "Stout, 307 Northampton Street, Easton, Pa." **192:** T. **193:** C; "Harris, Skaneateles, N.Y." **194:** C; "W. H. Brown, Jewett City, Conn." **195:** C; "W. Shaw Warren, Art Photographer, No. 29 Temple Pl, Boston, Mass." **196:** C; "J. H. New, Cohoes, N. Y." **197:** C; "Glines, Newton, Mass." **198:** T. **199:** C; "D. E. Pardee, Port Leyden, N. Y." **200:** C; "J. O. Durgan, Norwich, Ct." **201:** C; "Sherraden, No. 516 Broadway, Council Bluffs, Iowa." **202:** C. **203:** C; "Drew, Dover, N. H."; "Lovingly yours, Marnie." **204:** C; "Cady, 194 High St., Holyoke, Mass." **205:** V; "Photographic Studio of Geo. H. Leck, 283 Essex Street, Lawrence, Mass." **206:** T. **207:** C; "Kelly & Co, Moncton, N. B."; "Auntie and Uncle from Laura." **208:** V; "Chas. D. Holmes, Boston Gallery, 405 Main Street, Worcester, Mass." **209, 210:** T. **211:** C; "A. Bogardus, Sherman & McHugh, Successors, 11 East 42nd Street, New York." **212:** T; "Ocean View Photo. Car, Nantasket Beach." **213:** C; "C. T. Collier, Riverside, California"; "For Susie E. Pratt." **214, 215:** T. **216:** C; "Hardy, 493 Washington St., Artist Photographer, Boston, Mass." **217:** T. **218:** V; "Dunshee Artist, No. 3 Tremont Row, Boston. Duplicates can be had anytime within two years." **219:** T. **220:** V; "Photographic Studio of A. M. McKenney, 12 Market Square, Portland, Me." **221:** C; "Langley, Artist in Photography, Crosby Block, 780 Elm St., Manchester, N. H." **222:** T. **223:** C; "John A. Todd, Photographer, 318 & 320 J Street, Sacramento, Cal." **224:** T. **225:** C; "M. C. Nilson, 76 Pleasant St., Malden, Mass." **226:** C; "Taggard, Stevens Bld'g, Central Sq., Lynn." **227:** C; "J. K. Cunningham, Gouverneur, N. Y." **228:** V; "Photographic Studio of E. G. Goldsmith, 374 Main St., Springfield, Mass. Duplicates furnished at less rates." **229:** V; "Warren's Portraits, Cambridgeport, Mass." **230:** C; "Ward, No. Adams, Mass." **231:** T. **232:** C; "Biddle, 34 E. Main St., Xenia, Ohio   Duplicates can be had at any time." **233:** C; "Geo. H. Thompson, Orange, Mass. Duplicates can be procured at any time. Special attention given to all kinds of portraiture in crayon,

ink, oil or water color." **234:** C; "Brooks, 294 Washington St., Boston." **235:** C; "Claflin, 377 Main Street, Worcester, Mass." **236:** C; "From Weston the Photographer, Bangor, Me. Negatives Preserved for future orders." **237, 238:** T. **239:** C; "H. A. Smith, Photographer, Winchendon, Mass. Duplicates furnished at any time." **240:** C; "T. H. Hare, Art Photography, Hamilton, Mo. Negatives Preserved. Duplicates can be had at any time." **241:** C; "Gagen & Fraser, Toronto." **242:** C; "W. Gatt, Brattleboro, Vt. Duplicates furnished at any time." **243:** C; "From the studio of Demer's & Son, Art Studio, 314 Main St., Holyoke, Mass. Negatives kept. Copies can be had."

The 1890s

244: C; "Gurley, 128, 130 & 132 Genesee St., Next to the Bridge, Utica N.Y. We make a Specialty of the New Instantaneous Process. Fine work at reasonable prices. The negative from which this photograph was printed is preserved for further orders." **245, 246:** T. **247:** C; "Fred L. Davis, 352 Washington St., Boston." **248-251:** T. **252:** C; "Geo. W. Ames, Lynn, Mass." **253:** C; "Pettit & Dickerson, 381 George St., New Brunswick, N. J." **254, 255:** C. **256:** T. **257:** C; "Salisbury, 43 East Avenue, Pawtucket, R. I." **258:** T. **259:** C; "Chase, Extra Finish, 65 Railroad St., St. Johnsbury, Vt." **260:** C; "From the well known Photograph Gallery of W. H. F. Heath, Bradford, Ohio. All negatives from which photographs have been made will be preserved and filed away systematically, and duplicates of this or any other picture can be had at any time. Special attention will be paid to copying and enlarging old pictures to any desired size, which can be finished either plain, in Crayon, Pastel, Water Colors, India Ink or Oil, at prices as low as good work can be produced." **261:** T. **262:** C; " 'Aureole' cards. Patent applied for." **263:** C; "L. F. Bates, 303 Westminster St., Providence, R. I." **264, 265:** T. **266:** C; "—offolk, Michael, Nebraska." **267:** C; "I. L. Hammond & Co., 172 Lisbon Street, Lewiston, Me. Small photographs enlarged to any size. Negatives Preserved. Duplicates can be had at any time." **268:** C; "H. E. Strout, Home Bank Block, Brockton, Mass. Artistic Photography. Instantaneous Portraits of Children a Successful Specialty. Duplicates can be procured at any time." **269:** C. **270:** C; "F. E. Taggard, Currier's Building, 333 Union Street, Lynn, Mass. Take elevator. Instantaneous Process used. Duplicates at reduced rates." **271:** C; "Dunn, Ripon, Wis." **272:** C; "Rice, 311 Main Street, Worcester, Mass." **273:** C; "Harris & Greene, 230 Genesee St., Utica, N. Y." **274:** C; "E. A. Lynn, Photographic Studio, Successor to Davidson, 1108 Pacific Ave., Bernice Building, Tacoma, Wash. Negatives preserved." **275:** C; "Miles, 151 High Street, Holyoke, Mass." **276:** T. **277:** C; "Corbett, Augusta, Kansas." **278:** C; "Barentzen, Portrait Artist. Awarded diploma of honor and decoration. Studio—Garnet, Street, Malden. Duplicates at reduced rates." **279:** C. **280:** C; "A. W. & G. E. Howes, Photographers, Ashfield, Mass. Parties wanting more Photographs like this must give year and number as on this card. Be sure and give the number and year right. For 1896 No. 5259." **281:** C. **282:** C; "Dana, Cor. 14th Street & Sixth Ave., New York." **283:** C; "The Shorey Studio, Lynn, Mass." **284, 285:** T. **286:** C; "Boyer Bros, No. 1316 Tower Ave., West Superior, Wis." **287:** T. **288:** C; "Armstrong Studio, 13 Pleasant St., Portsmouth, N. H."